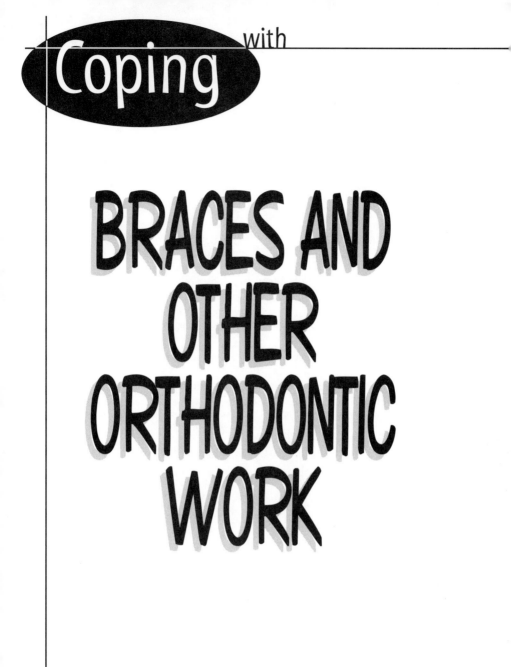

Coping with

BRACES AND OTHER ORTHODONTIC WORK

Jordan Lee

THE ROSEN PUBLISHING GROUP, INC./NEW YORK

Published in 1998 by The Rosen Publishing Group, Inc.
29 East 21st Street, New York, NY 10010

First Edition

Library of Congress Cataloging-in-Publication Data
Lee, Jordan.
    Coping with braces and other orthodontic work / Jordan Lee.
       p.   cm.
    Includes bibliographical referencces and index.
    Summary: Discusses why braces are needed, how to deal with den-
tists and orthodontists, the procedures behind orthodontic work, living
with braces and after, and dealing with the emotional side of wearing
braces.
    ISBN 0-8239-2721-0
    1. Orthodontics—Juvenile literature. [1.Orthodontics.]
    I. Title.
RK521.L44 1998
617.6'43—DC21

                                                            98-9276
                                                               CIP
                                                                AC

Manufactured in the United States of America.

About the Author

Jordan Lee is both a college instructor and freelance writer in Tulsa, Oklahoma. She contrasts her own experiences wearing braces in the late 1960s with her daughter's experiences now in the '90s. As she and her older daughter both suffer from TMJ, she has come to know a lot of dentists and orthodontists across the country.

Born and raised in New England, Jordan Lee now resides with her family near Tulsa.

Acknowledgments

Special thanks to Dr. James S. Torchia, D.D.S., M.S.D., who graciously shared his knowledge and expertise for this book. Dr. Torchia is a board-certified orthodontist who practices in Tulsa, Oklahoma. In 1993 he was named Oklahoma Dentist of the Year. Thanks, also, to his staff of dental assistants: Sherrie Hermann, Jeanne Keller, Sandra Hill, Jenni Ingram, Ellen Reynolds, and Kellie Brewer, who allowed me to watch them work and answered all my questions.

In addition, I'm grateful to the many persons who described their experiences wearing braces and retainers. Thank you, Jessica Clarke (an eighth-grader from Buxton, Maine), who comes from a family of braces-wearers: both her mother and grandmother wore braces as adults. Thank you, Nellie Clarke, for your stories, and to Michal Simpson and Melissa Young for their experiences.

Finally, thanks to all my students who volunteered their stories about the pleasure (and misery) of wearing braces. My book is more complete because of them.

Contents

Introduction:
Welcome to the World of Braces

Getting braces (or at least needing braces) is a common experience for American children. Ninety percent of you have crooked permanent teeth, and about 50 percent of you will obtain orthodontic treatment. Wearing braces isn't even a kids' event anymore; 20 to 25 percent of orthodontic treatment is devoted to adults. Why all this interest in braces and orthodontics?

The basic orthodontic techniques have been around for more than fifty years; the newer treatments are simply less conspicuous and easier to wear. Dental insurance has also made braces more affordable. In fact, wearing braces is such a common experience today that the social stigma once attached to it ("Hey, metal mouth!") hardly exists anymore.

Believe me, I can attest to the changes.

I got my braces in 1967. I always knew I would need braces sooner or later because of the space between my two front teeth, but I wasn't very happy with the timing of the event. I was in high school by the time my father (who didn't have dental insurance) had saved enough money to send me to the orthodontist, and I felt very self-conscious. I literally stopped smiling that year, and if I had to laugh, I put my hand up to cover my mouth. Furthermore, a mouthful of braces made dating and the goodnight kiss a dreaded event. Should I date a guy who had braces himself?

1

One thing that bothered me was that my braces didn't look like my best friend's. Her braces uniformly covered her teeth. My braces (because they were fixing a different problem, I guess) looked much different, as if the orthodontist had run short of metal bands and brackets: Some teeth had bands; some didn't. Where there were bands and brackets I had a hard time brushing my teeth, which meant I had to see my dentist more frequently (and I really hated my dentist). No matter how much attention I paid to my teeth, I kept getting cavities (which, of course, only worsened my fear of the dentist).

I wore those braces for two long years, getting them off just in time for senior portraits. And as far as my parents and I were concerned, the braces had been only for cosmetic purposes. It never occurred to me that braces were important for other reasons, such as correcting my bite so that my upper teeth didn't wear down my lower teeth. It never occurred to me that braces had anything to do with TMJ (temporomandibular joint syndrome) or even that I had TMJ (despite not being able to open my mouth wide enough to brush my emerging wisdom teeth). Back then, you got braces 1) if your family could afford them, and 2) if they would improve your looks. Nobody talked about muscle spasms, headaches, or periodontal disease. And nobody told me how biting your nails affected your teeth.

Twenty-five years later, my older daughter needed braces—not to improve her looks, but because her jaw kept locking. It was the first time I learned the connection between TMJ and malocclusion. My daughter's jaws were out of alignment, and braces would correct that.

I shuddered envisioning all that hardware on her teeth, but she seemed delighted with the idea of wearing braces and being like her friends. In fact, she actually enjoyed the experience (although the discomfort was still there). She even coordinated the colors of her elastic bands and ties. Clearly, wearing braces in the '90s is a lot different from wearing them in the late '60s. And dental insurance has made them a lot more affordable.

Until several years ago, no one apparently had thought to write a book about braces and orthodontia. Few books existed, although orthodontists and dentists kept pamphlets on the subject in their offices. If I had read one, I would have known to choose an orthodontist who would treat my TMJ as well as my looks. I would also have taken more seriously my habit of grinding my teeth and would not have ended up with a mouthful of expensive porcelain crowns twenty years later.

What happens with your teeth now directly affects your dental health years later. If you understand the importance of braces and a proper bite, you'll appreciate the miraculous changes your orthodontist can make: changes in your looks, how your jaws fit together, and how long your permanent teeth will last.

Why You May Need Braces

Shelly knew when she was in third grade that she would have to wear braces. Several of her permanent teeth had come in crooked, and when she smiled she showed a jagged row of teeth and empty spaces. Even at that age, she was embarrassed—she covered her mouth with her hand when she laughed and mumbled when she talked to avoid opening her mouth. Shelly was actually relieved when her dentist suggested she see an orthodontist.

Shelly didn't know much about braces or how they worked. All she knew was that people needed braces to make crooked teeth straight. If you asked her why she wanted straight teeth, she would have replied without hesitation, "I want to be pretty."

Improving your appearance is one of the reasons for having orthodontic work, but it's not the most important one. Preserving your teeth and the health of your gums, handling headaches and toothaches, and being able to chew food without pain are other reasons.

How can headaches and muscle pain be helped by braces? Before I can answer that, let's take a look at your teeth and their surrounding structures.

4

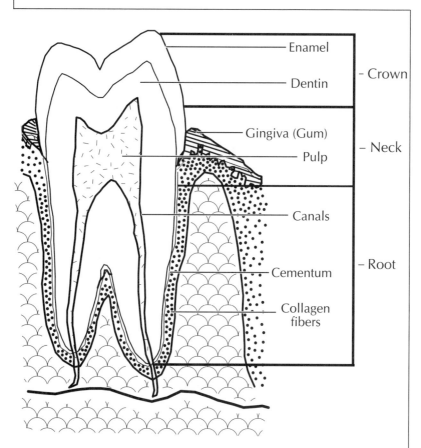

Parts of the tooth.

Anatomy of the Tooth and Jaw

A tooth is composed of several parts, and some parts are more sensitive to touch than others. Enamel coats the outside of the tooth; it's the hardest substance in the human body. Dentin lies beneath the enamel. When enamel wears away, the more yellowy dentin shows through. These two parts make up the crown of your tooth.

The pulp and root of your tooth extend down into the jawbone. Because the bone is pliable, teeth can be pushed and pulled into different positions. That's the purpose of braces: to push your teeth into better positions.

Your jaws are made up of two parts: the upper jaw and the lower jaw. The upper jaw is part of the cranium, the large bone that covers and protects your brain. Your lower jaw—what you actually chew with—is called the mandible. These two parts come together where the mandible meets the temporal bones (one on each side of the head at the temples). The temporomandibular joint is the point at which they come together. Your jaws can grow at different rates, and uneven jaw growth can lead to an underdeveloped lower jaw or an overhanging upper jaw. Because the upper and lower jaws are supposed to work together, it's important that they fit well together.

Take a look at your teeth. Your upper and lower teeth are supposed to fit nicely together (or else you won't chew your food well). Pretend to bite something. Do your teeth fit together like the pieces of a jigsaw puzzle, or do you have trouble making your upper teeth line up with your lower teeth? Uneven jaw growth can lead to bite problems, which then lead to chewing problems, muscle fatigue, and damaged teeth.

Why do so many people have bite problems? For one thing, evolution has created a few of them. As human beings have evolved, our brains have become larger and our jaws smaller. Since the number and size of the teeth have remained the same, some mouths are overcrowded. Our American heritage (meaning mixed ethnic heredity) also contributes to problems. What if you inherit your father's teeth (which happen to be larger than most) and your mother's jaw (which happens to be smaller than most)? Clearly, the combination will create an overcrowded

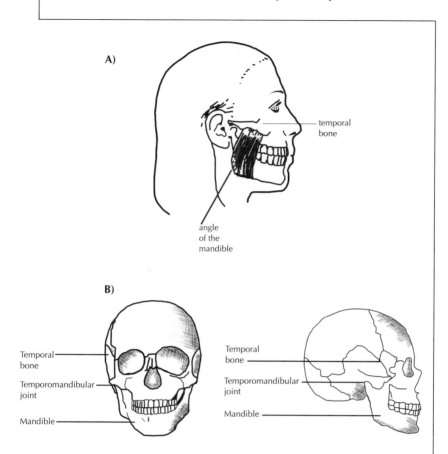

A)

temporal
bone

angle
of the
mandible

B)

Temporal
bone

Temporomandibular
joint

Mandible

Temporal
bone

Temporomandibular
joint

Mandible

(a) The strongest chewing muscle is the masseter, which originates on the temporal bone and inserts on the angle of the mandible. (b) The temporal bone and the mandible form the temporomandibular joint.

mouth. And an overcrowded mouth leads to crooked teeth, hard-to-brush teeth, and ill-fitting upper and lower teeth.

Specific Bite Problems

When the dentist talks about a normal occlusion, she means a normal bite. That's when the teeth in your upper and lower jaws fit together perfectly when you bite something. The teeth are straight and well spaced, with no gaps.

A Class I malocclusion is not very serious as malocclusions go. In this case, your jaws line up correctly and you upper and lower molars fit together, but you have crooked teeth.

A Class II malocclusion results when the jaw relationship is not equal. Your upper first molars are half a tooth or more ahead of your lower first molars, causing your upper jaw to stick out.

A Class III malocclusion results when your upper first molars are half a tooth or more behind the lower first molars, causing the lower jaw to stick out.

In addition, you can have an open bite, in which your front teeth don't meet when you close your mouth. As you can imagine, if your front teeth (upper and lower) don't come together when you bite down on something, you're going to have a hard time biting through food with your front teeth.

A closed bite causes a different problem: The teeth of the smaller jaw (usually the lower one) hit the gums of the other jaw instead of the teeth. Teeth biting on gums causes damage to the surrounding tissue.

In a cross bite, your jaws don't meet properly, from side to side.

Teeth need to fit together properly so that you can chew properly. If your teeth don't chew together, your jaws may ache.

Crowded and Crooked Teeth

Overcrowded teeth result when a mouth is too small, or when some teeth have come in after neighboring teeth have leaned into the available space. Overcrowded teeth affect your appearance, and they are hard to keep clean.

Flossing can be difficult—you succeed in wedging the floss between the tightly spaced teeth only to end up having the floss get stuck.

When flossing is so hard, people may stop doing it. But not flossing can cause even worse consequences for your teeth. Poorly brushed teeth collect bacteria and food debris, which combine with saliva to cause plaque. If plaque is not removed, minerals in the saliva cause it to calcify and turn into hard-to-remove tartar. Tartar may cause gums to become infected, which may lead to periodontal disease and deteriorating bone support.

Problems in Spacing

Spaces between teeth are common in children who lose their baby teeth before their permanent ones are ready to come in. If the space is not filled soon by the permanent replacement, nearby teeth lean into the open space. By the time the permanent tooth starts to erupt, it has lost its original space. Crowding and crooked teeth result when teeth have to compete for space.

Sometimes when the permanent teeth come in, there's a space between the upper front teeth. Braces can help close that gap, too.

Bad Habits

Bad habits are another reason you might need braces. Thumbsucking and tongue thrusting (pressing your tongue against your front teeth) are two bad habits that will misshape your teeth. Both affect your upper front

9

teeth, pushing them outward. If the habits are broken before the permanent teeth come in, the damage may be minimal. If the habits persist past the age of six or seven, you'll need braces to reposition your permanent teeth.

Biting your fingernails or sticking toothpicks or paperclips between your teeth are other damaging habits. These habits usually cause trouble with spacing and also wear down the affected tooth surfaces. If practiced long enough, braces are needed to correct the spacing problems.

Temporomandibular Joint Disorder (TMJ)

Most people can open their mouth wide enough to insert three fingers. I can only open wide enough for two. As a child, I hated going to the dentist because keeping my mouth open for such long periods made my jaw muscles ache. I often bit the dentist's fingers—I just couldn't hold my mouth open any longer. Had either of us suspected temporomandibular joint disorder (TMJ for short), we would have figured out earlier why this kept happening.

TMJ is a painful joint condition of the muscles in the face, neck, and upper back. Although TMJ cannot be cured, it can be treated, and one of those treatments calls for braces to reshape the jaw position.

The dentist had assumed that I refused to open my mouth any wider. The truth was I couldn't. My facial muscles were so tight from clenching my teeth day and night that they no longer permitted my mouth to open a normal amount.

Since about 50 percent of the population suffers from some degree of TMJ, you may want to see if it is contributing to your need for braces.

Symptoms of TMJ

The symptoms of TMJ mimic those of other disorders. A common symptom is headaches—the kind that occur mostly on one side of your face, particularly around (or behind) the eyes, cheeks, and temples. Pain is often referred to other areas, making it hard to detect the source. You might have a burning, tingling sensation in your tongue, frequent earaches, and sinus headaches that are not related to infection or congestion. You might have neckaches (because the neck muscles are attached to the facial muscles) or tenderness in your face.

TMJ can occur on one side of your face or both sides at once. You might notice a clicking or popping noise when you open or close your mouth. If the TMJ is severe enough, your mouth might lock in the open position.

Causes of TMJ

Usually there is more than one cause of TMJ disorder. Accidents account for many jaw injuries. Some injuries are direct, such as blows to the jaw (such as in fights or car accidents). Other injuries result from whiplash in car accidents in which you're jolted backward (or sidewise), and the pain or problems show up only months later. Sometimes one jaw grows faster than the other, causing trouble in closing the mouth.

Finally, bruxism (clenching or grinding your teeth) is a major cause of TMJ disorder. Clenching or grinding the teeth wears them down and creates malocclusion, or an unbalanced bite. Malocclusion affects the chewing muscles and puts stress on the joint where the mandible connects with the temporal bones. Let's take a closer look at the temporomandibular joint.

Parts of the Temporomandibular Joint

A smooth rounded protrusion lies on each side of the mandible at the joint. It's called a condyle, from the Greek word for "knob." The bony condyle needs a cushion between itself and the temporal bone it meshes with; otherwise bone would grind against bone. A specialized cartilage called the articular disc lies between the condyle and the temporal bone. Tough connective tissues attach the articular disc to the condyle, but sometimes the disc becomes dislocated, allowing the condyle to come in contact with the temporal bone. That's when problems begin.

Muscles are also an important part of the temporomandibular joint. You use several sets of chewing muscles: one set for opening the mouth, another for closing; one set to move the jaw forward, another to move it backward. If one set of muscles is overworked and fatigued, it affects the other muscles. The neck muscles and the upper back muscles are connected to the chewing muscles, so if your facial muscles are overworked, you can end up with an aching neck and back.

When you clench your teeth, you work the strongest chewing muscles, the muscles that attach the mandible to the temporal bone. These are in the area of the cheeks. If you have unbalanced muscles (because one set has been worked more than another), you risk stressing the joints and pulling the articular disc out of position with the condyle.

Direct blows to the jaw will also displace the disc and condyle, creating pain and difficulty in moving the jaw.

Diagnosing TMJ

How does a dentist know if you have TMJ disorder? One

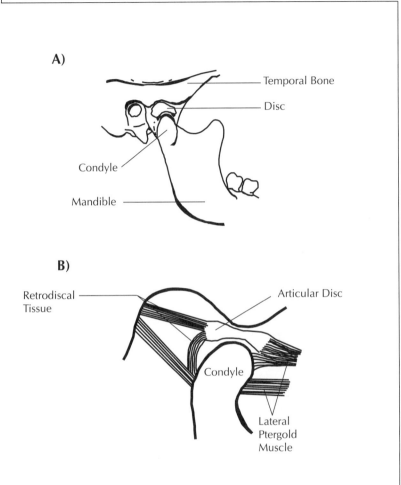

A)

Temporal Bone

Disc

Condyle

Mandible

B)

Retrodiscal
Tissue

Articular Disc

Condyle

Lateral
Ptergold
Muscle

(a) Parts of the temporomandibular joint. (b) When the mouth opens, the upper part of the
retrodiscal tissue stretches to its full length and helps stabilize the disk on the condyle.

who is familiar with the disorder can make a diagnosis
based on your symptoms. If you're not sure whether your
jaw pops or clicks when you open and close your mouth,
try this simple exercise. Insert your little finger into your
ear and then carefully pull the finger down toward your
chin. Keeping the finger in place, slowly open your
mouth. At some point, you may hear a slight popping

sound. Keep the finger in place as you slowly close your mouth. Listen for another popping or clicking sound.

Doctors can confirm the diagnosis by ordering a CAT scan. CAT stands for computer-aided tomography. The machine prints X ray pictures of the area scanned. It depicts the shape and condition of parts within the temporomandibular joint, specifically the condyle and articular disc.

A CAT scan does not hurt. It can feel a little strange, though; I felt as if I were being rolled into an oven, but it was completely painless. If you suffer from claustrophobia, you might discuss the procedure with the lab technician in advance, because you will be inside the machine for a few minutes.

Treatments for TMJ

There is no definitive cure for TMJ disorder; however, certain treatments are helpful in reducing its discomfort. Bruxism cannot be cured either, but dentists can minimize the damage done to the teeth. Learning relaxation techniques and reducing stress will help to reduce the amount of clenching you do when you're awake, but other methods must be used if you grind your teeth at night.

Dentists make nightguards out of hard acrylic to fit over either the upper or lower teeth. One kind, called a flat plane splint, fits snugly over the teeth, slightly separating the upper and lower teeth. The side facing the other teeth is flat and smooth, so that the opposing teeth slide over the surface when they come in contact with the splint.

The other kind of splint, called a repositioning splint, also fits snugly over one set of teeth; but instead of a smooth surface facing the opposing teeth, it has shallow indentations for the opposing teeth to fit into when the mouth closes. This splint gently forces the jaw into a new position as it protects the teeth from damage.

Nightguards don't stop the clenching, but they do prevent the wear and tear on the teeth. The nightguard may last from five to ten years, depending on how seriously you grind your teeth.

Heat and massage help to relax the muscles of your face, neck, and back. But you still need to correct the malocclusion that stresses the muscles, and braces may be the best way to do it.

Without Braces, What Might Happen?

Without braces to correct your bite, you risk fractured teeth (from constant wear and tear, as well as from an overbite that leaves the front teeth unprotected).

You can have speech problems, because your teeth affect how you pronounce certain words. If you figuratively "chew your words," you may do so because you're embarrassed by unsightly teeth or have trouble coordinating the movements of your jaws.

Without braces, you will wind up with joint problems affecting not only your facial muscles, but your neck and shoulder muscles as well. And finally, the quality of your teeth will decline.

The Most Common Time to Get Braces

Most problems are best treated after the permanent teeth come in. That usually occurs for girls around the age of eleven and for boys around thirteen. Some young people get braces much earlier, especially if the orthodontic work is done in stages. You may be given your first appliance or set of braces around the age of seven or eight in the hope that you may not need later treatment. Sometimes the braces may be removed and then reapplied a couple of years later when the rest of the permanent teeth have come in.

Dealing with Dentists and Orthodontists

David hadn't been to the dentist in five years, ever since his parents divorced when he was ten. His mother stopped making dental appointments because she no longer had insurance. David was relieved. He had always dreaded those visits to the dentist, and now he had an excuse not to go: He was saving his mother money.

David had a problem, though. He knew his teeth were not in the best shape. Some had grown in crooked, and he thought he had some cavities because he got toothaches when he ate sugary foods. On a weekend visit to his father, one of David's teeth started to act up. Drinking anything hot or cold made him yelp in pain.

"Better have that checked," his father said.

"Oh, it's done that before," David said, rubbing his hand over his jaw.

"What does the dentist say about it?" his father asked.

David tried to change the subject. "Where's the newspaper? Want to see a movie today?"

His father looked up. "What does the dentist say?"

"I haven't seen one in a while." David pretended to be looking for the newspaper.

"How long is a while?"

"A few years, maybe," David said, not looking at his father. *"Hey, I hear there are some good shows at the dollar movies."*

"Are you trying to change the subject?"

"I just thought we could go to the movies."

His father looked at him intently. *"You never did like going to the dentist,"* he said. *"Have you even seen one since I last took you?"*

David squirmed. *"No,"* he admitted.

"You haven't been to the dentist in five years?" he said.

"Well, Mom doesn't have dental insurance," David said.

"Tell her I'll pay for it. Then make an appointment. You don't want to lose your teeth."

"I brush them," David said. *"I'm not going to lose them."*

"Well, you've probably got some cavities, and besides, with your teeth crooked like that, I'll bet you need braces, too."

"I don't need braces," David said. His face paled.

"Just make that appointment," his father said. *"Better yet, I'll make the appointment."*

David thought for a minute. He didn't want to see the dentist. The last time he'd been there, he'd practically passed out listening to the dentist drill another patient's tooth in a nearby room. Just the whirr of the drill made his hands go cold and his heart start to pound. No, he definitely didn't want to go through that again.

"I've got soccer practice every day after school," David said. *"I'll make an appointment this summer."*

"No, you won't wait till summer," his father said. *"If your teeth are so sensitive to hot and cold, there's*

probably something wrong. Besides, you need to have them cleaned. I'll make an appointment for you during school hours."

"Well, check with me first; I might have a test that day."

"What's the deal, David? I'm offering to take you to the dentist and get you out of school for an hour or so. Since when have you been interested in taking tests on time?"

"They're hard to make up," David said, looking at his plate. He really wasn't good at lying.

"I'm still making that appointment, and I'll take you there myself."

The day of the first appointment, David was sick. He canceled the appointment. The second time, he simply "forgot" about it and went on a field trip. The third time, David's father made the appointment for first thing in the morning and had David spend the night before at his apartment.

As they drove to the dentist's, David sat glumly in the front seat. He gazed out the window, seemingly prepared to jump out of the car at the next stoplight.

"Stop wringing your hands," his father said. "Quit making this into an ordeal."

"I just don't think it's important," David said. "My tooth hasn't bothered me in a while."

His father parked the car. "Come on, let's get this over with."

David got out of the car and briefly considered running away. He was disgusted with himself. What was there to be afraid of? The dentist had stuff to give you so you wouldn't feel any pain.

But listening to the sound of the drill would make him sick. So what if he didn't feel the pain; he'd still be hearing that drill.

They got on the elevator. David refused to push the button to the eighth floor. "This is really silly," his father said, pushing the button himself.

At the dentist's office, David felt weak and trembly. He slowly followed his father into the waiting room. His hands were cold and clammy, as he absently flipped through a magazine.

A dental hygienist called David's name. David's heart threatened to explode. He briefly considered fleeing, then dejectedly followed the hygienist to her office.

As she tied a bib around his neck, David felt faint. I can't go through with this, he thought. I've got to get out of here. "I need to go to the bathroom," he said.

"It's right down the hall to the left," she said. "Are you feeling okay?"

"Not really," David said. He bolted from the room. Once in the bathroom, he threw cold water on his face. It's only a dental exam, he told himself. It's not going to hurt. I can do this.

Someone knocked on the bathroom door. "Hey, are you okay?"

David realized how silly this must look. How could he explain being fifteen years old and still afraid of the dentist? How would he ever get his teeth fixed?

When David opened the door, the dentist was standing there. "I think we should postpone this exam," he said, to David's immense relief, "and talk about what we can do to make this a better experience for you. Come on, we can talk in my office."

Fear of Dentists and Orthodontists

Believe it or not, David's experience was not unusual. Many people carry their fears of the dentist into adulthood. In fact, 75 percent of Americans have some fear of the dentist, and 10 to 15 percent are actually phobic about it.

A phobia is an exaggerated fear so intense that the person cannot control it. People may avoid the dentist for twenty years or more, until something becomes too painful to bear. Even then, they may be too upset to let the dentist do his job.

What could cause people to skip appointments and neglect their teeth?

People of your parents' ages who avoid the dentist probably do so because of unfortunate earlier experiences. In the 1960s and even into the '70s, dentists didn't have the best equipment to work with. Low-speed drills made cleaning out cavities an ordeal. Dentists were often reluctant to use enough novocaine or nitrous oxide to render the patient painfree.

And some dentists were like mine: unaware how to deal with the squeamish patient. Whenever my first dentist set out to drill a cavity, I would suggest a whopping dose of novocaine, and he'd say, "Oh, let's try it without novocaine first. If it starts to hurt, just raise your hand, and I'll stop drilling. Then we can see if you need a shot of novocaine."

In the beginning, I trusted that dentist to keep his word. Of course, I wasn't exactly a model patient. I interpreted every sensation as being painful. When he started to drill, just the sound of the machine made my heart pound. Maybe I only thought I was being hurt, but within seconds

21

I'd raise my hand and flap it around wildly. The dentist kept drilling until my behavior was too distracting. Then he'd stop and say these horrible words. "Just hang on a minute more. I'm almost done. You don't need novocaine now."

Well, I'd put my hand down, and he'd go back to drilling. Every time I'd raise my hand, he'd tell me he was almost done. And, of course, he was never done. He'd make my parents come in so I'd behave better, but it didn't bother me to act out in front of them.

Children who have bad early experiences with the dentist dread dental appointments because they expect more of the same. They don't know that the newer equipment makes drilling cavities faster and far less painful, or that nitrous oxide can render the patient so calm he doesn't care what the dentist is doing.

Maybe you fear the dentist because of your parents' earlier fears. If you fully expect a bad experience, you often get what you expect. If you've heard enough scary stories about the dentist, you will accept them without question. Or you watch how your parents handle their dental appointments and adopt their behavior. I have three children; the two youngest look forward to their dental appointments and lament that they can go only twice a year. My older daughter, however, reacts the way I do. She's always anticipating pain and discomfort. Why do they behave so differently? Could it have anything to do with the fact that their father (who doesn't mind having his teeth worked on) has usually taken the younger two to the dentist, and I always take our older daughter?

You may stay away from the dentist because you've been neglecting your teeth, and you don't want to hear a lecture about it. Perhaps you think the dentist will criticize you for having cavities or having so much plaque on your teeth that the hygienist has to spend the greater part of the visit removing it.

Charlotte hated going to the dentist for cleanings. She brushed her teeth diligently, but she couldn't get the hang of flossing. Besides, it took forever, and she was always too tired to floss before bed. Nonetheless, each time she went for a cleaning, the hygienist would mention that she hadn't flossed. "Here, I'll show you how to do it," the hygienist would say, handing Charlotte a mirror while she tore off a long piece of dental floss.

Embarrassed at the thought of a lecture, Charlotte would hold up the mirror to her reddening face. I won't go through this again, she would say to herself as she opened her mouth for the lesson.

Then again, you might fear dental appointments because you don't like the feeling of not being in control. When you're sitting in the dental chair, or the orthodontist's chair, you may feel at the mercy of the doctor. You don't know what he's planning to do next, and you don't know whether it will hurt. Even if the doctor says it will only hurt a little, how do you know that his "little" is the same as yours? Do you trust him to stop drilling when you ask him to? Do you know the alternatives to any painful procedures?

Perhaps you wouldn't mind the dentist so much if you didn't associated the sound of the drill with pain. To me, the sound of the drill is forever associated with pain (and a dentist who wouldn't quit when I asked him to, which is not even the case anymore).

Perhaps you're most afraid of the pressure of pulling and twisting that goes on when a dentist pulls a tooth or tightens braces. It can be easy to equate all uncomfortable sensations with pain. But pressure and pain are not always the same. Sometimes simply hearing the dentist murmur to his assistant can convince you that all is not going well. If you then expect pain, you'll probably feel it. Stress or fear actually excites the body and makes you more aware of your feelings. It's easy to mix up pain and fear and nervousness.

Those of you who are truly phobic and can't stand the thought of instruments or fingers in your mouth may need professional help to overcome your fear. Avoiding the dentist unfortunately only reinforces the phobia. The more you seek relief by avoiding (skipping and canceling appointments), the more frightening the dental experience will become. You may have suffered other early traumas that cause you to panic at the thought of someone working on your mouth. The only solution is to explore those traumas and work with a sensitive dentist or orthodontist who will respect your concerns.

Solutions to Your Fears

First of all, you need to realize that avoiding the dentist because of your fears only reinforces them and makes them grow. If you neglect regular cleanings, you risk the creation of larger problems ahead.

The first thing to do is to address your fears with your dentist or orthodontist (if it's the braces you fear most).

24

Make an appointment just to share your fears with the doctor, and then together plot a strategy to work through them. Sometimes it's enough just to let your dentist know what worries you. In my case, if the dentist tells me ahead of time what to expect and describes what he's doing along the way, I don't become so anxious. I do not handle surprises well, so if I know what to expect, I'm much less fearful. Maybe that's all you need.

Work out a signal to cue the dentist when you need a break. Make sure the dentist is willing to stop when you signal. Of course, if you signal every few minutes, you can't complain when your appointment takes longer and you are charged more. But having a signal that your dentist will follow gives you back some control.

Ask a lot of questions. Make sure you know what each procedure is like. Most patients, I'm told, don't ask enough questions. You have the right to know exactly what your dentist intends to do when making an impression of your teeth, for example. You have the right to know what alternatives exist for pain control. You have the right to decide how much pain you can handle. Both a novocaine shot (which numbs the area in which it's given) and nitrous oxide (otherwise known as laughing gas) make formerly torturous experiences painfree. Nitrous oxide has the added benefit of calming the patient who is nervous about dental treatment.

Other Ways to Cope

Relaxing
Perhaps you don't think relaxing and dental visits go

together, but you can learn to relax so that your mind doesn't interpret every sensation as painful. The first step is learning to recognize when you're tense, so that you can let go of the tension. Progressive muscle relaxation helps you relax, but you can't practice it only in the dental chair. You need to practice tensing and relaxing all your muscles once or twice a day. There are many good books on progressive relaxation techniques. All encompass the same principles: Isolate one set of muscles, tense them and hold for a count of five, then relax for a count of five.

You can start anywhere you like and work down or up your body. I usually start with my hands. I tense my hand by balling it into a tight fist. I hold that tension while I silently count to five, then I open my hand and try to let it go limp. Next, I do the same thing with my forearm, trying not to involve my hand or the upper part of my arm. I tense only the specific muscles I'm working on. Isolating the muscles is the hardest part, but it's important to learn how to keep the rest of your body relaxed even when one part is tense.

Tensing and relaxing all the muscle groups (from your facial muscles all the way to your toes) should take about thirty minutes. The idea is to recognize when you're all tensed up so that you can release that tension. Tense muscles make everything hurt more; that may be one reason why you think you experience so much pain.

Another way to relax is to concentrate on your breathing. Breathe through your nose. Mouth-breathing can lead to hyperventilation, and when you hyperventilate, you increase your anxiety. Breathe in slowly to a count of

26

three, hold for three seconds, and then exhale to a count of three. If you focus on this pattern, your brain will be too busy to notice other distractions.

Learning to tolerate discomfort (or to reinterpret the feelings) can raise your pain threshold as well. If you're at the dentist's or the orthodontist's and you start to feel pain, first try to observe the sensation. Pretend you're a reporter and your job is to describe this particular feeling. You may discover that it's discomfort rather than pain. The more objective you can be about it, the more you learn to tolerate.

Of course, if the pain really bothers you, ask for something to stop it. Know what options exist for pain management. Just remember to relax your mouth if the dentist gives you a shot of novocaine. Tensing for the needle only makes it harder on you. The dentist may apply ointment to numb the area where you'll get the shot. While you'll still be able to feel the needle, it won't hurt as much.

Listening to Headphones

If the sound of the drilling bothers you most, take headphones with you and listen to soothing music. Many dentists keep headphones for patients, but if yours doesn't, just take your own. And there's no law that says you must listen to soothing music. Perhaps heavy metal would distract you better from the sound of the drill. Maybe an audio tape of the latest bestseller would be more distracting for you. The point is: If outside noises cause you distress, make yourself unable to hear them.

Tranquilizers

Dentists and orthodontists prefer not to prescribe tranquilizers for teenage patients for a couple of reasons. For one thing, tranquilizers reinforce the patient's belief that he can't handle the appointment on his own. Relying on a pill for relief makes it easier to count on the pill for the next visit. More important, though, tranquilizers are addictive. Taking an addictive substance in your teen years could lead to abuse in later years.

Handling the Gag Reflex

Some people gag more easily than others. Maybe you're one of those who gag when the dentist tries to make an impression of your teeth. Overcoming the gag reflex is really very simple: Just breathe through your nose. Even if your mouth is full of plaster, your nose is free. If you concentrate and breathe through your nose, it will slow your breathing as well, ultimately calming you. If you keep telling yourself not to gag, however, your mind is so focused on that possibility that you end up doing what you least want to do.

Desensitization for Phobics

If you are one of the 10 to 15 percent who are phobic about the dentist and orthodontist, you may want to use a desensitization ladder to learn to overcome your fears. The ladder is imaginary; you'll be visualizing it. On each rung you imagine a different fear. The higher you climb, the more intense the fears. For example, if you're afraid of having your teeth drilled, you might start by imagining the dentist's waiting room. That's the bottom rung of the ladder. If you're phobic, just that may make you nervous. When you start feeling anxious, visualize a different, more peaceful scene. As you start to relax, return to the image of the dentist's waiting room.

Keep switching back and forth between the two scenes until you can remain comfortable imagining the waiting room.

When you've conquered that particular fear, you take another step up the ladder. This time, visualize the assistant ushering you down the hall to the dentist's office. As you start to feel nervous, imagine the peaceful scene. Keep switching back and forth until you can comfortably tolerate visualizing that walk down the hall.

Your next worst fear may be sitting in the dentist's chair. Apply the same procedures to help you grow comfortable with that image. On you go up the ladder, encountering more intense fears. Once you can visualize yourself having a tooth drilled and not complaining, you can test your fears in the real world. It may take several months before you're desensitized enough to handle actually going to the dentist, but you can conquer your fears this way. Have a friend help you, to remind you to stay calm and visualize your peaceful scene. You can learn to tolerate your fears and rise above them.

Selecting an Orthodontist

How should you choose a dentist or an orthodontist? Today, because many insurance companies have a specific list of doctors to choose from, you may not have much choice. But talk to your friends about their practitioners. Find out what they like or dislike about them. You'll want a dentist with whom you feel comfortable because you'll always need to see a dentist to have your teeth cleaned. If you have a dentist and need braces, the dentist will probably recommend an orthodontist. Ask for more than one referral so that you can choose for yourself one who will meet your needs.

Any orthodontist you consider should have a D.D.S. or a D.M.D. after his or her name as well as a license to practice dentistry in your state. In addition, your orthodontist should have completed a full two-year postdoctoral program in orthodontics in an accredited university. Also helpful, but not necessary, is knowing whether or not he or she belongs to the American Association of Orthodontics and is board-certified or a Diplomate of the American Board of Orthodontics.

How will you know these things? If certificates are not displayed around the office, ask. You have a right to know his or her qualifications.

In addition to qualifications, however, you'll want to know if he or she has the necessary skill and is personable enough that you'll want to visit every month for the next two or three years. Word of mouth can tell you if an orthodontist is competent and personable, but you also need to judge for yourself. Make an appointment to interview the orthodontist. Ask questions about his or her plan for your mouth; ask how many people he or she has successfully treated. You can usually tell how you would get along with a doctor by the end of the first visit.

Meanwhile, take a peek at the office and dental assistants. Here are some things to look for.

⮑ Do they seem competent and pleasant?

⮑ Are they stressed from too many patients?

⮑ Do they sterilize their equipment after each use?

⮑ Do they wear gloves when putting their fingers in your mouth?

⇝ Do they change these gloves after each patient?

⇝ How do they interact with each other?

Let your parents know ahead of time the qualities that mainly interest you. Even if your insurance company has only a few doctors it recommends, you should consider them all. Of course, the cost is something that will interest your parents. Orthodontic treatment today can cost more than $3,500. You'll want to make sure your orthodontist has reasonable rates compared to others. It's certainly okay to ask him or her how much everything will cost and whether you can set up a payment plan in case your insurance doesn't cover all of it.

Before Getting Braces

Your dentist who recommends that you get braces will tell you why you need them. The orthodontist can go into more detail after he has taken some X rays and made an impression (called a plaster study cast) of your teeth. X rays are not painful, but some can be uncomfortable. Having an impression made is another standard procedure. The dental assistant mixes up some powder and liquid to make a gummy substance that she puts in a mouthpiece. She then inserts the mouthpiece over your teeth. She will do only one set of teeth (uppers or lowers) at a time. When the plaster starts to harden, she wiggles it a little to loosen it from your teeth and then removes it.

The whole procedure is painfree and quick. If you're worried about gagging, remember to breathe through your nose. On occasion, bits of the plaster have fallen down people's throats, but you're not likely to choke on the little that gets loose. It's sometimes flavored with cinnamon or peppermint, so it's not unpleasant. By the time your orthodontic work is finished, you should be a pro at having impressions made.

Your orthodontist will use the X rays and plaster study cast of your teeth to determine the exact problem and how to correct it. Believe it or not, he does have a plan for fixing your teeth, and you have a right to know that plan each step along the way. If he intends to use certain appliances (explained in the next chapter), you certainly should know why he's using them.

Some teenagers think it's impolite to question a doctor, who is supposed to know what he's doing. However, it's not impolite to want to know 1) what is wrong with your teeth; 2) how braces or other appliances will remedy that problem; and 3) how best to take care of your teeth while you're in braces. If you are well informed, you will probably realize the importance of following the doctor's directions. And that will make your experience of wearing braces that much more successful.

If you're still nervous about any procedures, ask if you can watch the doctor work on a few of his patients. The more familiar you are with the procedures, the more comfortable you will be. Most orthodontists will have no objection to your watching them work, as long as you don't get in the way.

Just remember, although your parents most likely are footing the bill or splitting it with the insurance company, you should have a say about the orthodontist you're using. After all, you're the one who is most directly affected.

The Basics of Braces

The good thing about braces is that they're a noninvasive technique (meaning that your skin is not punctured or cut) to reposition teeth and jaws. Novocaine is not required, because the orthodontist does not touch the sensitive parts of the tooth (the pulp or root). The most you will feel is a dull ache from the initial pushing and pulling on your teeth.

Components of Braces

Braces are called fixed appliances because they are attached to your teeth. Some appliances that are described later in this chapter are removable, but the braces themselves (unlike retainers and headgear) cannot be taken out of your mouth whenever you want. The orthodontist or dental assistant will take them off when the time is right.

A generation ago metal bands were attached to most of the teeth, but now bands are placed only around the back teeth or those supporting headgear or hooks. Instead, brackets are bonded right to your teeth or onto the bands you do have. Brackets can be steel or ceramic. Some are even clear to be less conspicuous. The problem with them, however, is that food may discolor them.

The brackets are the pieces to which the archwire will be attached. Archwires come in various thicknesses.

Treatment usually starts with the thinner wires and gradually moves on to the thicker ones. The thickness of the wire correlates with the force needed to move a tooth. The thicker the wire, the stronger the force exerted. The brackets and bands are merely supporters for the archwire; it's the job of the archwire to move the teeth. The orthodontist shapes the archwire into a U to conform to your mouth. He bends and snips the wire to make it fit your mouth. You'll have two wires: one covering the top teeth, and one covering the bottom teeth.

The dental assistant wraps tiny plastic rings around the bracket to hold the archwire in place. These come in different colors, so you can coordinate your rings with the season's colors or your team colors. The rings are changed each month along with the archwire, so you can change the colors every month.

The bands on the back teeth may have hooks for headgear, for rubber bands, and to hold the end of the wire. If the orthodontist needs to exert more force to pull teeth together, he may use a continuous elastic chain, attached from one faraway tooth to another.

If you've lost a baby tooth too early and the permanent one is nowhere in sight, your orthodontist may have you wear a space maintainer. Space maintainers do just what you'd expect—they fill the gap to hold the space open until the permanent tooth comes in. Without a space maintainer, the teeth on either side of the empty space would start to lean in on the gap. Then the permanent tooth would come in crooked. Some dental assistants slip rubber tubing over the archwire where a space maintainer is used because the wire has no tooth to lean against.

A)

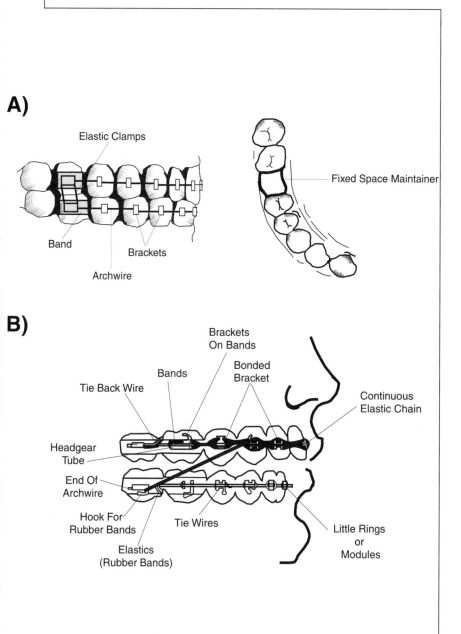

Fixed orthodontic appliances.

Some people choose to get inside braces. With these braces, the brackets are bonded to the inside of the teeth. They are less visible but reportedly take longer to achieve the same results as outside braces. They also cost more.

Additional Appliances

Some of you may need additional appliances with your braces. One common appliance is the palate spreader, which is used to gradually widen the roof of your mouth. Several conditions make this appliance necessary. If your bite is off, widening the roof of your mouth allows the upper teeth to mesh better with the lower teeth. If your mouth is overcrowded, widening the palate provides more room for all those teeth. Finally, if you have trouble breathing because of a high palate and narrow arch, the palate spreader will widen the air passages.

The orthodontist cements the palate spreader into place, attaching it to the back teeth. In the middle of the roof of the mouth is a joint that allows for separation. When the palate spreader is activated, it gently pushes apart the roof. Eventually, as the palate expands, bone fills in the space to make the wider palate permanent. You activate the palate spreader twice a day, placing a key in a hole in the center and turning it until the next notch shows in the appliance.

The palate spreader may be a little uncomfortable when first activated, but it won't hurt. You may feel the pressure of the teeth being pushed apart, and you may notice a space between your two front teeth. Don't worry; that space between will fill in. After the palate spreader has done its job, you'll leave it in place for a while longer until new bone has had a chance to grow.

The Herbst Appliance

Your orthodontist may decide to use a Herbst appliance to move your chin forward in order to improve your bite. As you can see in the diagram, the upper jaw is connected to certain teeth in your lower jaw. The rod and plunger attached to the lower teeth fit into the tube or sleeve that is attached to the upper molars. Screws that stick out hold the rod and tube in place; thus you may find that your cheeks are a little irritated at first because of the screw heads rubbing against them.

Headgear

Most of the teens I spoke with said that wearing headgear was the worst part of having braces. It wasn't that the headgear hurt; it merely embarrassed them because it was so conspicuous. That 's the bad news: being conspicuous. The good news is that you don't necessarily have to wear your headgear to school. You put it on when you get home, and you sleep in it. Headgear may only need to be worn for twelve hours a day.

Headgear comes in different types because it treats different problems. As you can see from the following diagrams, headgear may only cover your mouth and extend back to your neck. More elaborate headgear covers the top of your head in addition to the back of your neck. It depends on where your orthodontist needs to exert the most force.

The purpose of headgear is to improve the direction of your facial growth. With all headgear, you'll have a wire face

Screw Head

Metal,
Acrylic
or Plastic
Bonded To
Your Teeth

Screw Head   Rod or   Tube or
                  Plunger   Sleeve

The Herbst appliance.

bow consisting of an inner bow and an outer bow. The inner
bow inserts in your mouth and attaches to your braces. The
outer bow attaches to the inner bow and extends around your
face to the safety strap in back. Depending on whether your
orthodontist wants to pull your teeth back or up and back,

38

he'll use either a regular type of headgear or a "high pull." Sometimes, a combination is used.

If you require headgear at any time during your treatment, be sure to ask your orthodontist to explain what he wants to accomplish with it. Then follow his instructions about wearing the headgear (anywhere from twelve to twenty-four fours a day). If you're not consistent about wearing it, you'll simply prolong the time you have to be in braces.

The easiest way to keep track of the time spent wearing your headgear is to keep a chart. Copy the chart below and record the number of hours you spend wearing your headgear. Keep a weekly tally, and be honest with your orthodontist. He will suspect something if you swear you wear it fourteen hours a day when you're barely getting in three hours every other day. Owning headgear and actually wearing it correctly are two very different things.

The Process of Having Braces Applied

Having braces put on is usually a two-day process. Most people don't have both upper and lower braces applied at the same time; it takes too long. So be prepared for two visits. For some of you whose teeth are quite close together, the orthodontist may use an additional appointment to insert separators between your teeth. These small pieces will push your teeth apart just enough that bands can be placed around them without too much discomfort. When the orthodontist puts on your braces, he'll remove the separators.

In larger offices, dental assistants do a lot of the setup work for the orthodontist. You'll first become acquainted

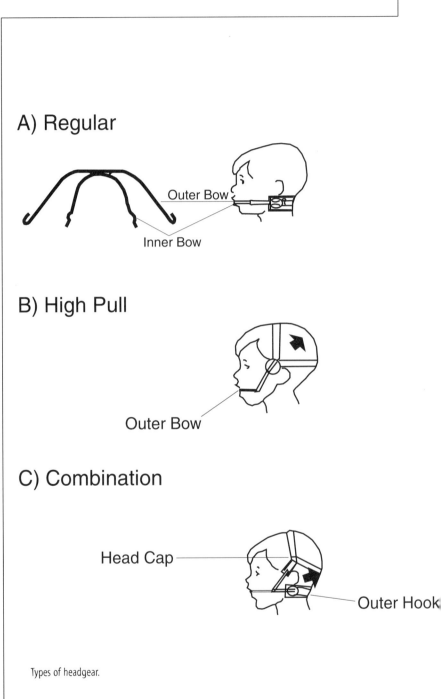

A) Regular

Outer Bow

Inner Bow

B) High Pull

Outer Bow

C) Combination

Head Cap

Outer Hook

Types of headgear.

with the mouthpiece that holds your mouth open and keeps your lips from touching your teeth. It's important to have your teeth perfectly dry when applying glue and brackets. This particular mouthpiece feels uncomfortable—especially for those who can't open the mouth wide—but it doesn't really hurt.

The other equipment you'll see on the dental stand are scraping tools, different sizes of pliers, a suction hose, mixture for glue, and a spectrum curing light that may look like a handheld hairdryer. Scraping tools are used to scrape away excess glue on the teeth. The orthodontist needs a perfectly clean tooth surface to work on. The dental assistant uses different sized pliers to attach the tie rings to the brackets and archwire. She uses the suction hose to keep your mouth dry; if she needs to rinse your mouth, she'll use the suction hose to draw out the liquid, including any saliva that may have accumulated. The glue is

	Sunday	Monday	Tuesday	Wednesday	Thursday	Friday	Saturday
Time Spent In Headgear							

Sample chart for wearing headgear.

often a mixture of powder and liquid. The assistant mixes the potion just before the orthodontist is ready to glue the bracket to the band or tooth. The spectrum curing light shines a bright light that dries out the area. This speeds the drying time, helping the glue to set faster.

If a dental assistant is working with the orthodontist, her job will be to clean the surface of the teeth, preparing them for the braces. She'll mix the glue and prepare the bands, brackets, and archwire. The orthodontist will do the actual bonding of the brackets to your teeth. She decides the placement, and she'll cut and shape the archwire to fit your teeth, although the assistant may finally insert and attach the archwire.

The Importance of Asking Questions

You may be a very inquisitive person, but if you're like the majority of other patients you probably won't ask many questions about what's happening in your mouth. Josh is a typical example. As I stood by to watch him have his braces put on, the dental assistant arranged the tools to work on Josh's teeth and then mixed the glue.

Josh lay back in the dental chair. He grimaced when she inserted the mouthpiece that stretched his mouth open and pushed out his lips.

The dental assistant went right to work, cleaning and drying his teeth. She laid the bands and brackets out on the tray for the orthodontist, who was slipping on a pair of gloves. Josh stared out the window.

The orthodontist patted his arm. "You feeling okay?" he asked.

Josh nodded, but his look said, "Hurry up and get this over with."

The orthodontist picked out a band and wiggled it over a tooth. When he was satisfied with the fit, he slid it off and let the dental assistant add some glue. Then he molded the band to the tooth.

When all the brackets had been bonded to the teeth, the orthodontist cut and shaped the archwire. He handed it to the dental assistant and pulled off his gloves. "You're almost done," he said to Josh, who was still staring out the window.

Before the assistant attached the archwire, she asked Josh what color tie rings he wanted. Josh shrugged and indicated he didn't care.

"Well, then, let's put you in blue," the assistant said, reaching for the plastic tie rings. She expertly attached them with her tiny pliers. When she was done, she handed a mirror to Josh.

He barely looked in the mirror, as the assistant started telling him when and how to use wax and how to floss with the special thicker floss she handed him. Josh said nothing. He merely took the floss and packet of wax and jammed them into his pocket.

"Do you want some Tylenol?" the assistant asked.

"No, thanks," Josh said, as he got up to leave.

"Are teenagers always this quiet?" I asked the assistant.

"Most of them are quiet and uncomplaining," she said. "It's the adults who question every move I make, or complain that the mouthpiece is uncomfortable."

"I guess you must be relieved that you don't have to explain everything," I said.

"Actually, it's better when they ask questions," she replied. "Patients need to know what their braces are supposed to be doing. They need to know what to do if some part breaks or comes off. They should know when a situation is a real emergency and they need to call us.

"I try to think of all the questions they could ask, and answer them, but sometimes I forget to tell them certain things. One kid thought the wire that kept scraping his cheek was supposed to be like that. His whole cheek was cut and bleeding by the time of his next appointment. A little bit of wax would have helped him."

The point of this story? It's perfectly okay to ask questions at the orthodontist's. He or she will be glad to explain procedures and purposes, because an informed patient is usually a more compliant patient. And the more you consistently follow the expectations, the faster your braces will do their job.

The Fun Part of Braces

Playing around with colored elastics and tie rings is the fun part of braces. You can pick out colors to match the holidays or to match your team if you play sports. Usually the first thing the dental assistant asks when you come in for your monthly appointment is, "What colors do you want this time?"

The bright colors are most noticeable in the first few weeks of wear. After a while the colors fade or become discolored by food or drink. By the time you hardly notice them, it'll be time for a new set.

A word of caution, though. Listen to the dental assistants when they tell you that certain colors don't wear well. If you go with clear tie rings (and most dental assistants advise against them), realize that the rings will turn the color of your food and drink. Colas will turn them brown; mustard will turn them an unsightly orange. Black tie rings can make you look as if you have a mouthful of cavities.

Problems While Having Braces Applied

Having braces applied is not really an ordeal; you may encounter problems, but few are serious. You may be surprised at the resilience of your teeth. All that prying and pushing may seem to loosen your teeth, but they won't fall out. Teeth are supposed to feel loose because they're being moved to new positions, but they won't become so loose that they break or come out when the orthodontist attaches bands and brackets.

What's the likelihood of swallowing a bracket before it is glued into place? Dental assistants tell me that patients have swallowed all kinds of little pieces of braces without any harm. If something slides down your throat, it will eventually pass through your system. Swallowing hardened chunks of glue may feel funny, but it won't hurt you.

Does it hurt when the braces are attached? Most adults I spoke with said the process didn't really hurt. Some didn't even notice any discomfort until a few hours later. What you probably *will* notice, however, is the pressure on your teeth and the dull ache from teeth being pushed into different positions. Sometimes, the orthodontist doesn't clip the end of the archwire close enough, so a little piece irritates your cheek. He can fix that if you point it out in time. If you don't notice it until after you go home, you can put a tiny ball of wax over the protruding wire until you get back to his office.

Years ago when I got my braces, I felt discomfort rather than pain. My teeth felt heavier with all that metal surrounding them, and I couldn't keep from running my tongue over all the parts. The rough places bothered my cheek, and wax didn't seem to help much. I was always afraid I would swallow the wax or accidentally spit it out when I was talking. Now, I have to admit it didn't hurt to have the braces attached. But an hour or so later, my mouth ached, and my teeth felt tingly. And all that metal in my mouth was unpleasant. Fortunately, taking Tylenol and ibuprofen reduces the discomfort even better than prescription pain relievers. Many orthodontists suggest taking the medication before your appointment and continuing it for several hours afterward. If left untreated, the discomfort can turn into a headache.

Your teeth will probably be sensitive for a few days. If you try to bite into something, that may hurt, because your teeth are temporarily sensitive from the added weight of the metal and the pressure of the wire. As odd as this sounds, some people have gotten through the first days of sensitivity by mashing their food against the roof of the mouth with their tongue. It was the only way they could chew. Other people stuck to liquids and soft foods until their teeth stopped tingling.

Some teenagers told me a different story. Janice, who is fourteen, said that it hurt to get her braces on. "My teeth and gums throbbed for three days," she said.

"Well, I'll admit your teeth probably ache, but that's not to say the whole procedure hurts," I said.

"That dull ache hurts," Janice said. "I couldn't eat for days."

"And Tylenol and ibuprofen didn't do that much for the pain," her friend assured me. "Boy, I thought the orthodontist was going to break my teeth apart with all that pounding and gluing. My teeth sure were sore. Don't you call that pain?"

"Well, I said your teeth would feel sensitive,"I replied, looking over my notes.

"I lost ten pounds when I got braces because I couldn't eat anything good,"Janice said. "You better tell people it does hurt."

"I guess it boils down to what you consider hurts."I said. Nonetheless, if it'll add another dimension to my book, I'll write that many teenagers felt it hurt to have their braces attached."

"Well, just say it was unpleasant,"Janice suggested.

"And it's more of a dull ache that lasts a while,"her friend added.

The truth is that people have different thresholds of pain awareness. Relative to other dental work, having braces put on doesn't hurt that much. But some teenagers equate dull aching teeth with intolerable pain. If you go in expecting a bad experience, you may have your expectations met. Better to anticipate an easy time.

Length of Time in Braces

You will probably wear your braces for six to twenty-four months, although thirty months is not unusual. It all depends on the nature of your problem and how well your teeth respond to the braces. If you're supposed to wear additional appliances but don't wear them faithfully, you'll probably have to stay in braces a lot longer.

When the orthodontist calculates how long you'll have to wear braces, she's assuming you will be a compliant patient. Noncompliance always lengthens treatment, so it's best to be patient and try as best you can to cooperate.

Now that you have braces, what can you expect? Obviously, your life will change somewhat: You'll be visiting the orthodontist every month, you'll have to avoid certain foods, and your teeth will feel conspicuous and fragile when playing most sports. The bad news is: This will probably last two years or more. The good news is: You'll get used to the changes in time, and the end result (straight teeth) will be worth it all.

Appointments with the Orthodontist

The major difference between seeing an orthodontist with a large practice and one with a small practice is which one actually works with you more. In a large practice, the orthodontist employs one or more dental assistants who do a lot of his setups and changing of archwires. Don't worry; the orthodontist always tells them what to do and then checks their work. In a smaller practice, the orthodontist does all the work himself. Sometimes an orthodontist practices as both orthodontist and dentist. At separate appointments he cleans your teeth, fills cavities, and adjusts your braces. What's the best way to go?

You have to decide what is more important to you. If you're interested in building a relationship with your orthodontist, you may not like spending much of your appointments with his assistants. However, whether he does the work himself or oversees his assistants, the quality of the work should be the same.

On the plus side, dental assistants may seem less intimidating than the orthodontist, so you may feel less foolish complaining to them about any discomfort.

Living with Braces

No matter what, though, you'll be seen every four weeks for adjustments to your braces. The archwire and the ring ties (that hold the archwire in place) are changed each time. Sometimes problems crop up during treatment that you didn't have before. For example, one of my daughter's front teeth started to turn sideways midway through her course of treatment. Her orthodontist must have anticipated that movement, because he didn't seem surprised but started work straightening the tooth after his other work had been done. Sometimes addressing one problem creates another.

What both surprised and reassured me was that an orthodontist has probably seen all the dental problems that exist. And he has a plan for correcting each one. Originally I thought an orthodontist decided each month what needed to be done, attacking each problem as it arose. Later I learned that an orthodontist has treatment strategy. That's where the plaster study cast comes in.

The orthodontist studies the plaster cast to determine the extent of your problems. Then he follows a plan of treatment based on what has worked in the past for others with your particular problems. In other words, he knows from the outset what he plans to do, or he knows what he has to do based on how your teeth respond to treatment.

Appointments are not all the same. Some may be longer because the orthodontist has to add more brackets or make another impression. Usually, you'll know ahead of time if the appointment is to be a long one. The dental assistant will tell you what the orthodontist plans to do, so you can tell the person who schedules your visits.

You can either schedule your appointments around school or during school hours. If you're seen during school, your orthodontist will sign a slip indicating that you've been at a dental appointment. School administrators will consider that a medically excused absence. Some kids prefer not to miss school for appointments, so they make theirs for after school. Dental offices are more crowded at those hours, but they will try to accommodate your particular needs.

Keeping Appointments

It's important to keep regular appointments. Skipping or postponing appointments affects your progress. Your orthodontist has calculated the length of your treatment based on your being seen every month. If you're seen on an irregular basis, your archwires will stay in one position longer than necessary. Skipping appointments is also inconsiderate to your orthodontist, who has set aside that time to see you. If you don't give twenty-four-hour notice of cancellation, some orthodontists will charge you for a "no show."

Be sure to bring with you any headgear or other removable appliances. The orthodontist needs to check their fit and make any necessary adjustments.

One teenager told me that she ate a breath mint before her appointment, thinking the minty odor would make her teeth seem cleaner. The orthodontist took one look at her mouth and said, "Well, you didn't clean your teeth very well. There's a residue all over them."The girl was too embarrassed to admit she'd eaten a mint instead of opting to brush her teeth before the appointment.

At many offices, the dental assistants instruct you to brush your teeth before appointments. They even give you a new toothbrush each time and little sample packets of toothpaste. Dental assistants and orthodontists don't need your breath smelling clean when they work on your braces, but they do need all the food and debris cleaned from your braces. You don't want them to remove your archwire and see clumps of lettuce between your teeth. You might feel embarrassed at first, standing in front of a communal sink and brushing your teeth, but once you realize that everyone is doing the same thing, it becomes part of the routine.

Regular Appointments with Your Dentist

Speaking of cleaning your teeth, you'll need to see your dentist more often than usual. That's because it's harder to keep your teeth clean when you have braces. Food that lodges between your teeth will decay and lead to cavities. Plaque builds up faster when brackets and wires are in the way. Consequently, dentists schedule more frequent checkups to keep your teeth healthy during this time.

You can make the dentist's job easier if you spend extra time caring for your teeth. The orthodontist can recommend special floss designed for use around braces. The floss is thicker in the middle than regular floss. Each end of the thread looks like plastic string, which enables you to insert it more easily between your teeth and the metal brackets. Then when you pull the floss through, the thicker part collects any debris and pulls it out as well. Flossing regularly will keep plaque and tartar to a minimum.

Using a Water Pik is helpful, too. A Water Pik shoots a stream of water at your teeth; the power of the spray dislodges any food or debris and washes it out. Electric toothbrushes may make brushing more appealing, but there will still be many places hard to reach because of the braces. The danger, of course, in not cleaning your teeth properly is that food that gets stuck between your teeth can go unnoticed and cause decay. Paying closer attention simply means brushing and flossing after eating.

Watching What You Eat

Certain foods will be off limits as long as you have your braces. Hard candies can break the brackets right off your teeth. Brackets bonded directly to your teeth may look neater, but they're actually more fragile. You also have to be careful when chewing raw vegetables. And it's nearly impossible to bite into an apple without snapping off a bracket.

Likewise, you'll want to avoid chewy foods, like caramels and taffy. Chewy stuff will pull off the brackets and wires. Hard, sticky candy tugs on your braces, just as bready food sticks to your teeth and wires. Biting into a fresh bagel has also been known to damage brackets.

Some orthodontists permit you to chew sugarless gum, but many frown on any gum, period. The chewier the gum, the more likely it is to pull out parts of your braces. To be safe, gum is better left out until your braces are removed.

You may be discouraged upon hearing all the great stuff you can no longer have. Some of you won't notice until you've had your braces on for a while, and suddenly you start craving hard or chewy candies. Some of you might not even be interested in eating when your teeth ache in the beginning, but eventually most people become acclimated and don't go hungry. If your teeth hurt too much for you to eat solids at first, try eating soups, Jello, and puddings. (My mother's favorite treat was a coffee milkshake.) Your teeth won't hurt the whole two years, and you'll soon graduate to regular food.

When my daughter started missing caramels and gum and popcorn, I suggested that she make a list of all the things she was going to eat when her braces came off. She kept updating the list as the months rolled by, but eventually she only truly missed gum.

Try not to give in to your urges to eat forbidden foods. Even though the orthodontist can always repair damaged brackets or bands, it prolongs treatment. Often you crave certain foods only because they're forbidden. Get your mind on something else, and you'll forget you think you can't live without popcorn.

Dealing with Problems

Sore teeth can be a big problem, but it's a fixable problem. The first few hours after an orthodontic appointment, your teeth may be sore. Sometimes that can even last a few days, but taking ibuprofen and acetaminophen will reduce the pain and inflammation. Rinsing your mouth with warm salt water will reduce swelling. If you usually have sore teeth after a visit, try taking the ibuprofen and acetaminophen an hour before your visit and continue through the day. Plan little treats for yourself and you may notice the pain less.

Don't confuse loose teeth with sore teeth. Often after an appointment your teeth will feel loose. But they won't fall out. The whole point of braces is to move your teeth around, so it makes sense that your teeth will loosen up at times. That will stop once the jawbone tightens around them. Mention your concerns to your doctor, but loose teeth are not usually a sign of disaster.

Breakage

Despite all your good intentions, you can still wind up with broken brackets and loose wires. Even if you're to blame for some breakage, don't try to hide the fact from the orthodontist. If a loose wire is cutting your cheek, cover the end with a ball of wax; you can get a supply from your orthodontist or buy some at the drugstore. The wax protects your cheek from the abrasive wire until the orthodontist can snip the wire or take it off.

If you snap off a bracket, check to see if the archwire is still being held in place by other brackets. If that's the case, save the bracket that fell off and take it to your next appointment, so your orthodontist will see what's missing. If a band (the metal piece that surrounds your tooth and supports other structures) breaks, it may be more serious. If the archwire seems to rely on this band for support, call your orthodontist and report what's wrong. He can then advise what to do next. If it's bad enough, he may schedule you for an emergency appointment.

If something you're eating gets stuck in your teeth, and you're afraid you can't remove it without pulling out the brace along with it, call your orthodontist for advice. It might help to try flossing first. But if you seem to be dismantling the braces, call your orthodontist right away.

You should also call your doctor if your gums seem infected, especially if you're running a fever. You may not want to call the orthodontist in the middle of the night (if you're not in too much discomfort), but you won't want to wait a couple of weeks for your next appointment, either. As a rule, infections don't clear up by themselves. Sometimes food has lodged under a wire and decayed, causing problems in the gums as well as the tooth. Prompt attention will lessen your discomfort.

If you're hesitant to call your orthodontist, err on the side of caution. Call and speak with a dental assistant to determine if the problem needs an unscheduled visit. If she suggests another course of action, try that first. She'll let you know how serious the problem seems to be.

What to Do When You're Out of Town

If you're at home and lose a band, you can always call your orthodontist. But what if you're visiting your grandparents in another state, and something goes wrong with your braces?

Whenever you're planning an out-of-town visit, check ahead of time for available orthodontists in the area. Ask your orthodontist what credentials to look for, and under what circumstances to call someone.

If something happens, you'll know when to call the local emergency room and when to make an after-hours call to a local orthodontist. Always carry your own orthodontist's telephone number with you. An emergency room doctor may want to confer with him or her if you've been in an accident and your braces are messed up.

The Danger of Braces and Sports

A lot of parents think braces and sports can't go together. But try telling an athlete she can no longer play softball or soccer until she gets her braces off. Most will find ways to keep playing.

Actually, braces present a hazard whether you're playing the game or simply watching it. My daughter was watching a friend play basketball just after she'd got her braces. At one point, my daughter ducked a ball that was thrown into the stands. In the process, her brace caught on her lip. She couldn't even holler because the snagged brace kept her lips from opening. Grabbing a pocket mirror, she finally figured out how to untangle the wires and lips. She wasn't hurt so much as embarrassed, because the crowd found her behavior more entertaining than the basketball players. The point of this story is that injuries can happen whether you're on the court or not. Prepare by taking precautions.

Types of Accidents

Soccer, hockey, basketball, and of course, football seem to be the most dangerous sports for people with braces. That's because the ball (or puck) is always flying around, and players have little or no protection for their faces.

As a soccer coach, I've seen more than my share of mishaps. When you're watching teenagers play soccer, you know you'll see about half of them in braces. One season, the goalie on my daughter's team finally got her braces off. She had a beautiful smile. Her mother, though, made her wear a huge plastic mouthguard "to protect that smile." Lisbeth objected strenuously to the mouthguard, but the day she took a flying soccer ball full in the face, she was grateful for the protection. Her face stung from the blow, and her teeth rattled, but the mouthguard kept everything in place.

Mouthguards

Speaking of mouthguards, they have disadvantages as well as advantages. The chief problem is that you can't readily communicate with one in place. If you've ever watched a basketball or soccer game (or played in one), you know that all the players talk to one another. "I'm open," "Watch your on-sides," "Shoot," "Pass it back." Now, wear a mouthguard that fits over your teeth and braces, and try shouting commands.

Kids tell me the mouthguards make them drool and mumble. In extreme cases, mouthguards make it hard to breathe when you're running. Because of these problems, some kids opt not to wear their mouthguards, risking damage to their teeth and braces.

However, mouthguards do a great job of protecting your teeth. If you get injured, you won't additionally cut your lips and cheeks or swallow parts of your braces. Dental assistants tell me they can adjust your mouthguard if you're having trouble breathing. "It's a matter of poking more holes in it," one told me.

As for the difficulty in talking, work out other ways to communicate with teammates. Hand signals work when teammates are close enough; otherwise, devise a system of hollers and grunts to signify what you want. In the middle of an important game, players don't speak in elaborate sentences anyway.

Headgear

Never wear headgear when playing sports! The refs probably wouldn't let you on the field or court anyway, but wearing external appliances is asking for trouble. Headgear is fragile, and sports can be high-impact. Aside from ruining expensive orthodontic appliances, you risk greater personal injury. Imagine some player grabbing your outer bow and yanking on it. Imagine yourself on the bottom of a pileup and someone's hand twisted around your safety strap at the back of your neck. Imagine getting tackled and landing on your face. Some sports may be off limits to you when using headgear. Whether you've taken the headgear off or not, the sport may be just too dangerous. In less strenuous sports, you might get away with playing without your headgear.

The Problems with Injuries

For your parents, the main problem with injuries (assuming you're not seriously hurt) is the expense of repairing any damage done to your teeth and jaws. Putting on new brackets and bands is one expense, but correcting your jaw's misalignment is even more costly (in time as well as money). Your short-term complaints may be cut cheeks and lips and sore teeth, but these are actually minor compared to jaw dislocation. A case in point:

My daughter Stevie had finally got out of her braces after two and a half years. Her dad and I had just finished paying for those braces a week before one of her roughest soccer matches. "I'm glad she's got the braces off," I said to her dad, thinking that at least she wouldn't cut her lips on metal if she fell down.

When Stevie went into the game, she overheard one of her opponents whisper to another to "take out #16." Since Stevie is tall and sturdy, she didn't think anything would come of the threat. But knowing that she was her team's best shot, she figured the opponents would try to hit her.

Minutes later, Stevie kicked the ball downfield just as two opposing players sandwiched her, sending her to the ground. Stevie landed right on her face, having had no time or room to put out her hands to break her fall. The ref blew his whistle, acknowledging the foul. Stevie's dad was screaming for a yellow card.

Stevie pulled herself up, holding her jaw. "Oh, no," I thought. "All that dental work, and she's probably broken her jaw!"

Stevie's head was swimming, and she came off the field. Later we called the orthodontist because Stevie's jaw had started popping and locking open once again.

The orthodontist agreed to see her the next day. Stevie had indeed knocked her jaw out of alignment. Even though she was in retainers at the time, the orthodontist made a splint to fit over her upper teeth, which would help the jaw settle back into place. If the splint had not done its job, the braces would have had to be replaced to correct the misalignment.

The danger of complicating your orthodontic problems or cutting the inside of your mouth is always present when you choose to play sports while wearing braces. A mouthguard lessens the danger, but nothing can protect you one hundred percent. However, many sports lead to injuries, whether the player has braces or not. Legs are broken, ankles sprained, and arms fractured. Injuries are just part of the risk of engaging in sports.

In short, you don't need to stop all your activities, but you do need to weigh the risks and take your own protection seriously.

The Emotional Side of Wearing Braces

Many teenagers are excited about getting to wear braces. "I finally feel like I'm fitting in," one teenager told me. "Everyone wears braces," another girl said. "I couldn't wait to get them on," added another.

Perhaps it's the excitement of something new; perhaps it's feeling more like the crowd. In any event, braces are extremely common, and most people initially are pleased to get them.

But there's a down side to wearing braces. The physical discomfort is one thing; I discussed that in chapter 4. In this chapter, let's consider the emotional side of wearing braces.

Sharla had been excited about getting braces because three of her friends had them, and she felt left out of their discussions. However, once she had them on, she realized that the experience was quite different from what she had expected. For one thing, the braces hurt. She called her friend Joan. "I thought you said the pain didn't last long," she said.

"Well, it didn't with me. Or, at least, I don't remember it hurting much; that was a year ago," Joan said.

"Well, I'm not going to choir practice tonight because my teeth hurt," Sharla said. "Singing might take your mind off them," Joan said.

"I don't want anyone to see me yet; I look stupid."

"What do you mean, you look stupid? Is that how you think I look?"

"No, you've been in braces a year, and I hardly notice the silver. It's just that my braces are so conspicuous," Sharla said.

"Oh, you'll get used to that," Joan said.

"That's what everyone says, but every time I look in the mirror, all I see is a mouthful of silver."

"So, quit looking in the mirror."

"That won't help. I'll still know that everyone can see them."

"Look, Sharla, people will notice when you first start talking, but after a few days nobody will think twice about them."

Sharla just couldn't see anything positive in wearing braces now. She didn't have crooked teeth; her jaw just needed moving. Her headaches were pretty bad, but how could the orthodontist be so sure that braces would stop them? She'd been excited about the braces until they were put on. Now she just wanted them off, or to hide out for the next year or two.

At school the next day, Joan ran up to Sharla with a bunch of their friends. "Okay, let's see how they look," she said.

Sharla reluctantly showed her teeth. "Hey, I like those colors," one girl said.

"Do you have to wear elastics?" another asked. "It's a real pain putting on elastics all the time."

Sharla felt a little more at ease since most of the group wore braces, too. She felt as if they were all part of a unique club. In fact, Sharla started feeling better about wearing braces. Until fifth hour.

This guy she liked sat across from her in math class. She kept wishing he'd ask her out. But with a bunch of wire around her teeth, she felt self-conscious.

Tony leaned over and whispered something funny about his last class. Sharla started to laugh, and without thinking raised her hand to cover her mouth.

By the end of the week, Sharla had acquired the habit of covering her mouth when she laughed and looking downward when she talked.

Nervous Habits

Thinking everyone is looking at you when you first wear braces is a common experience. You notice them because your mind is on them. And it's true that colored elastics and tie rings stand out when you laugh or talk. However, as common as braces are today, they don't carry the stigma encountered decades ago.

Kids will notice your braces and probably will remark about them, but that doesn't mean you should live in isolation for the next two years. Some people think up ingenious ways to cover their mouth when they talk. Others have tried talking without moving their lips much so that the braces won't show. Doing that leads to mumbling and having people ask you what you're saying. Maybe you'll just quit talking as much, nodding silently to your friends instead.

Hiding your teeth is not much of a remedy. The more you act embarrassed about braces, the more interest you'll inspire in them. People are always curious about things you want to keep hidden.

A better response might be to acknowledge that you're now wearing braces and accept that people will notice and comment at first. You're going to be in braces for a while. But if kids tease you about your braces, take it in stride. Agree (to some extent) with them, and then change the subject. Try to be nonchalant about your teeth so kids won't notice that they're a sore spot.

> *"Hey, John, let's see the teeth."*
> *John looks unperturbed. "What for?"*
> *"Hey, I like that sparkle," Sam says, obviously needling him.*
> *John looks up from his textbook. "They do shine, don't they?" John says.*
> *"Have you kissed anyone yet? I bet that's quite an experience."*
> *"What makes you say that?" John asks.*
> *"Oh, come on, I bet you'll cut their mouths up."*
> *"You got any advice on how to kiss a girl with braces?" John asks.*
> *"Well, it depends on if she has braces, too," Sam says, warming to the subject.*

Next thing John knew, they were off on a tangent, discussing Sam's advice about kissing. His friend had forgotten that he'd wanted to tease John about his braces.

The point is that people will notice your braces and no doubt comment on them. Pretending nothing is different doesn't work, because it will be obvious once you open your mouth. However, if kids try to embarrass you, try not to overreact. Many may simply be curious; talk matter-of-factly about the braces and all the good things they'll do for your teeth and appearance.

Sometimes acknowledging your discomfort will prompt others to take a different view, eventually comforting you about the experience. As soon as kids get used to seeing you in braces, the novelty wears off. You won't stand out anymore.

Problems with Braces

Wearing braces can sometimes create problems, but most are easy to deal with. Consider some of the more common experiences encountered.

Catching Your Braces on Your Lips

My daughter had this experience more than once, usually while she was playing a sport. All of a sudden, you are hit in the face with a ball going ninety miles an hour, and your brace catches and gets stuck on your lip. The problem isn't so much that the brace cuts your lip, as that it becomes *attached* to your lip.

If you panic, and my daughter did that only the first time, you'll hurt yourself. Instead, use a mirror so you can see how to pull the wire off the lip. Lips bleed a lot, even when the damage is minimal, so don't worry about the blood. If you break a wire in the process of getting it off your lip, call your orthodontist. Meanwhile, put some wax on the end of the wire. As for your lip, rubbing an ice cube over it will stop the bleeding.

Since braces can easily catch on your lips when you're playing sports, it's a good idea to keep a mirror and wax handy. Make sure your water bottle has enough ice in it to use on your lips in emergencies.

Although sports pose the biggest problem, sometimes your wires get stuck on your lips when you're not doing anything in particular. This happened to my daughter's friend in high school.

During math class, Melissa started chewing on her bottom lip in frustration over the assignment. Suddenly, her lip hooked onto the wire on her upper brace.

Melissa tugged on her lip, but it wouldn't unhook from the wire. She tried to wiggle her finger between her lips, but her lip was firmly attached to her top brace.

With a red face, Melissa walked to the front of the class. She leaned over the teacher's desk to ask permission to go to the nurse's office, but she couldn't speak clearly.

"What did you say?" the teacher asked.

"Can I have a pass to go to the nurse?" Melissa tried again to say, but her words were lost behind her lips.

"What's wrong with your mouth?" the teacher asked.

Melissa tried to show her, but of course couldn't move her lip. She stood there, feeling embarrassed.

Not knowing what was wrong, the teacher wrote Melissa a pass—for the *principal's* office.

Food Caught in Braces

Getting food caught in your braces doesn't necessarily hurt. That's the good part. The bad part is that if the food doesn't bother you, you may not realize it's there.

Several kids told me they'd gone to school with food hanging off their braces. One girl was so concerned about that happening that she brushed her teeth diligently before leaving home. More than once, she went to school with toothbrush bristles caught in her braces.

All that metal and wire in your mouth can easily snag some unsuspecting piece of lettuce or beef. With luck, you feel the discomfort of the lodged food, but that doesn't always happen. To be safe, you should always brush your teeth after eating. You can carry a toothbrush and travel-size tube of toothpaste in your bag to school or work. After lunch, take a few moments to check your teeth in the mirror and give them a thorough brushing. If you spot something that brushing won't dislodge, use dental floss to remove it. You'll feel more like smiling if you're confident that you don't have food caught in your wires.

Eating in Public

Try not to focus on food sticking in your braces; it doesn't always happen. However, there are things you can do when eating in public to keep problems to a minimum. First, choose soft foods, which won't cling so easily to your braces and teeth. Avoid salads; the raw vegetables can break brackets, and the lettuce can get caught around your wires. Substitute soup for salad. You can also break off brackets by biting into hard rolls.

If you choose your food wisely, you don't have to worry. After eating, go to the restroom and brush your teeth. If you didn't bring along a toothbrush, rinse your mouth with water and inspect for food particles. Use one of the toothpicks available at most restaurants to dislodge anything you see.

Unruly Elastics

Some people have to wear elastic bands on their braces in addition to the brackets and archwire. Elastics exert more pressure on the teeth and therefore can speed up the process of repositioning.

Here's the problem as I see it. We're not talking about huge rubber bands; we're talking about little tiny elastics. If you have trouble handling small things, as I do, these elastics can be a challenge. The orthodontist doesn't put on the elastics and expect them to stay there until your next appointment. Elastics are meant to be changed whenever you eat or brush your teeth, or if one breaks. I was amazed to see how easily my daughter and her friends put on an elastic and popped one off.

"That is truly impressive," I said. "I know I'd have trouble trying to hook that little thing around my teeth."

My daughter and her friends laughed. "Well, you don't always do it right the first time."

"Oh, you mean you get frustrated spending an hour trying to hook the elastic on?" I asked.

"No,"Allysha said. "But sometimes I've been trying to put one in, and it's popped out right onto the teacher's desk. Talk about embarrassment!"

Sindy laughed. "That guy in seventh hour finally asked me to sit with him at lunch. When I tried to remove my elastic to eat, it popped out right into his plate."

"Well, I swallowed one once. It snapped, and next thing I knew it had slid down my throat."

Everyone, it seemed, had a funny story to tell about their elastics. They soon became experts at putting them in and popping them out, and everyone apparently survived their mishaps. The best advice I got was to put them on in private; that way, you don't risk their flying off into someone else's lap.

Kissing

No doubt you've heard stories about people getting their braces caught on someone else's braces when they kissed. Most of these stories are just that: made-up stories. You can kiss without entangling your braces, although you won't want to engage in any deep kissing if you both wear braces. The wires are securely attached to your brackets with tie rings or something similar. They aren't hanging loose waiting to catch on someone else's brackets.

If you're wearing headgear, you're not likely to feel like kissing someone whether he or she has braces or not. In fact, I don't see how kissing is possible with an inner bow attached to your teeth and an outer bow hooked to a strap around your head. If you're going on a date and think you'll likely kiss the girl, take off your headgear and leave it at home. Braces alone will not be a problem.

Bear in mind, though, that if a loose wire is cutting into your cheek, chances are it will cut into your partner's if you attempt to kiss her before fixing it.

Wearing Headgear in Public

Not everyone who wears braces has to wear headgear, and not everyone who wears headgear has to wear it in public. Most people are told to wear their headgear ten to twelve hours a day, and that can occur during homework and sleep time. Headgear is conspicuous. If you have to wear it in public, some people may stare. Others may ask pointblank what it is and why you have to wear it.

Teenagers don't like to stand out; most want to blend in. Knowing this about teenagers, orthodontists don't expect them to wear headgear in public unless there are serious reasons. Some orthodontic problems may require twenty-four-hour wearing of headgear.

If you have to wear headgear in public because that will shorten the overall time you'll spend in braces, accept it. The first few times you venture out in public, you will probably feel embarrassed and conspicuous. If people stare at you, try to be matter-of-fact. Laugh if you can; you'll find that a sense of humor goes a long way toward making everyone more comfortable.

Develop some standard lines to answer typical questions. "This headgear fits on my braces and will eventually change the growth of my jaw." (This is the serious response.) "No, I'm not from outer space even though I may look like it. Believe me, I really can't fly." (The comical response.) "No, this stuff doesn't hurt, but the way people look at me does." (The putdown.) "I know this looks funny, and I wish I didn't have to wear it." (The genuine response.)

Think up your own comments, but sometimes the best response is none at all. In other words, ignore the looks. People will stop staring when your headgear becomes commonplace to them.

If you have to wear headgear, you have to wear it. If you don't make a big deal out of it, others probably won't. And soon enough, you won't have to wear it anymore.

Sleepovers and Headgear

Wearing headgear only at night is usually no problem unless you've invited someone over for the night, or you're invited to a sleepover yourself. Use your judgment. If it's only one night, your orthodontist probably wouldn't object if you skipped the headgear when you had a friend over. However, if you're going to visit a friend for a week, that's too long to leave the headgear behind.

It's helpful to talk openly about wearing your headgear at night. Don't make a big deal out of it; simply tell your friend or her parents that you have to wear this device that attaches to your braces. You may discover that people are curious about it, not frightened. Even your friend's kid brother may be interested in seeing how it hooks onto your braces and how the strap wraps around your head.

Braces and Photos

When I wore braces, I avoided getting in front of a camera. Pictures were never kind to me, and my mouth full of silver came off looking like blackened teeth.

But both photography and braces have come a long way since then. Many teens I spoke with hardly thought twice about having their picture taken.

"I wouldn't want my senior portrait done when I wore braces, but regular pictures don't bother me," Sharon said.

"I liked having pictures of me smiling in braces," said her fourteen-year-old friend, Sindy. "I want to remember what I looked like then."

"I was so proud of my braces, I always worked my way into photos," Rhonda said.

When my daughter first got her braces, we took close-ups of her teeth to send her grandparents, who live in New England. Stevie wanted them to witness her going from a mouthful of silver to a mouthful of straight, perfectly spaced teeth. Whenever she had her picture taken, she always smiled broadly for the camera. In fact, I have a picture of Stevie and her best friend, Amanda, at the time. They were leaning against each other, head to head, grinning big silver smiles at the camera.

Confident people smile with the mouth open. Braces are so commonplace that most teens don't mind having their picture taken. In fact, some people first start smiling with their mouth open when they're in braces, knowing that their teeth are being repositioned.

Making a scene because you don't want to be in a picture, or covering your mouth with your hand will only draw attention to you. Not smiling at all to avoid showing your braces makes you look unhappy.

My daughter's orthodontist used to send his patients to Glamour Shots to have pictures made once their braces came off. Glamour Shots is a photo studio that does a makeover before the photo shoot. Everyone apparently feels, and as a result looks, gorgeous. Then the orthodontist would hang his patient's favorite photo on his office wall to show others how well braces had worked.

Eventually most people get tired of wearing braces even if they were excited about getting them in the first place. Some people get tired of the monthly appointments; some get tired of not being able to chew gum or caramels. Some people are just ready to see their teeth again. The last few orthodontic appointments are "the best of times and the worst." If your progress is slower than your orthodontist predicted, you're bound to be disappointed. Unfortunately, he or she can't predict how fast your particular problem will respond to braces.

But finally one month you'll hear the orthodontist say, "Next month your braces come off." Teens reported mixed feelings when getting that news.

"I was so happy to get them off that I made a calendar of the last month," one girl said. "I crossed off the days like a countdown—seven more days till my braces come off. Three more days. One more day."

"I had a list of all the things I was going to eat once I got those braces off," another person said. "I brought a pocketful of change to the orthodontist's for that last appointment; I intended to go right out and buy the stuff on the way home."

"I was excited about getting them off," fifteen-year-old Donna said. "But the night before that appointment, I felt kind of sad. Like I was losing something. I'd been in braces for almost three years; I wasn't sure what I'd be like without them."

"I was ecstatic when my doctor said I'd get my braces off," Joshua told me. "But I have to confess, I was a little worried about the process. I mean, they'd used glue to put them on in the first place. How easy was it going to be when they tried to take them off?"

"I was happy to be getting mine off. It was time; all my other friends had theirs off, and I was beginning to feel that something was wrong with me because I still had mine on."

"How did I feel about getting the braces off?" one patient asked. "Relieved. Finally I was going to feel my teeth again."

"I was happy, too," Georgeanne said. "But I didn't tell any of my friends because I didn't know how I'd look and I didn't want an audience for that last appointment."

My daughter's friend Allysha summed it up best. "I couldn't wait to get my braces off," she said. "Overall, it had been a good experience. I'd bugged my parents to let me get braces in the first place, and I did everything (well, almost everything) my doctor told me to do. My headaches had stopped, and I was just ready to get this metal off my teeth. As far as I was concerned, the work was finished. I wanted to party when my doctor said I could get them off."

When the Braces Are Removed

Soon enough, the braces will have done their job, and your teeth will be repositioned. Now the orthodontist says your braces can come off.

Great Expectations

Most teens are ready to have their braces off, no matter how happy they were to get them in the first place. Everyone expects to look different—better—now that their teeth are straightened or repositioned. And everyone *will* look better, of course, or the orthodontist wouldn't remove the braces.

How you react when your braces come off depends to a large extent on your expectations. It's reasonable to expect your teeth to look straighter or closer together. It's reasonable to expect your facial shape to be changed as a result of the jaw repositioning. It's reasonable to expect to be happy with what you see.

It *isn't* reasonable to expect your whole life to change. You are not going to be more popular or a better athlete simply because your braces are off. Sports may be less of a hassle because you no longer have to worry about cutting your lips on your wires, but you won't necessarily turn into a spectacular athlete overnight. And you probably won't be the life of the party if you weren't when you were wearing braces.

If your life changes dramatically as a result of getting your braces off, it's probably because your self-esteem has grown. If you're suddenly more popular with your peers, it's probably a reflection of your new-found confidence. If you become a better athlete, it may be because you're concentrating harder on your play than on protecting your mouth.

Braces by themselves do not hold a person back. But how you feel about yourself while you're wearing those braces might. If you've been shy the whole time, you won't suddenly become a party animal. Apparently, that's not your nature. But being shy and then becoming more talkative when you're confident that you have a pretty smile is certainly possible. How you feel about yourself shows. Once your braces are off and you see how great your teeth look and feel, you'll no doubt look and act more confident.

Removing the Braces

The orthodontist may decide to remove your braces all at once or to remove one set (say, the top brace) and leave the other on a little longer. It has to do with timing; sometimes the upper brace has done its job before the lower brace has, or vice versa. Having one brace done at a time may be disappointing if you were expecting to get rid of all the metal at once, but you'll be a pro at the removal process when the other brace is ready to come off.

Despite your braces having been glued to your teeth all those months ago, it won't be difficult to remove them.

After all, remember how easy it was to snap off a bracket when biting into an apple. The time involved varies, depending on how many bands were bonded to your teeth and whether or not you're having both braces removed. Figure four hours for both. (Since that's a long time to spend sitting in a chair, you might consider bringing headphones to listen to music. My sources told me that the worst part for them was the boredom.)

The dental assistants usually get the job of removing braces and cleaning the teeth. The orthodontist with a large practice examines their work at the end. The assistant snips off the tie rings and pulls out the archwire. Then she uses a metal instrument to pop off the brackets. They're easier to remove than the bands, which are bonded to your teeth. Nonetheless, all the metal and ceramic is fairly easy to remove.

Once the metal comes off, the dental assistant must clean the tooth surface, as glue and debris will remain. Sometimes your teeth will be stained from the braces, but the orthodontist can help you take care of that. The scraping and cleaning take the longest time, and your jaws can get tired from keeping your mouth open so long. Most dental assistants will give you breaks to get up and walk around or use the bathroom. If she doesn't suggest a break, ask if you can have one when it's convenient for her.

Teenagers tell me that the process doesn't really hurt, but again, it depends on what you perceive as painful. You will feel pressure as the braces are being removed, but you should not feel any pain. You might feel as if the orthodontist is about to break your teeth, but that won't happen. Teeth are very resilient and movable. They will actually be a little loose when everything is done, but in a few days they will feel normal again. Your teeth have already been through a lot; they can handle being pushed and scraped one last time.

When the dental assistant and orthodontist are done, they'll probably suggest that you brush your teeth yourself to rid your mouth of any leftover cement. Here's your first glimpse of your new mouth. You'll notice how much easier it is to brush now and keep your mouth clean. You'll probably smile a lot in mirrors just to get used to those pretty white teeth, and you'll probably keep running your tongue over the smooth surface. Enjoy the experience; you've earned it. Wearing braces for a year or two was hard work, and now you're done.

Well, you're not totally done. If your orthodontist stopped right there, your teeth would soon move back to their old positions. Now he or she has to make retainers for you to wear twenty-four hours a day to "retain" the new positioning. About 95 percent of the correction he has made can be retained as long as you wear your retainer as directed. The average patient needs to wear retainers (upper and lower) for eighteen months to two years. But the process isn't as bad as it sounds.

Impressions

After your braces are removed, the orthodontist will make another impression of your upper and lower teeth. From this mold, he makes your retainers. (Often, this is a specialty for one of the dental assistants.) You'll be a pro at having impressions made of your mouth by that point.

The good part is that the dental assistant (or orthodontist) needs time to make the retainers, so you'll go home that first day with nothing on your teeth. You can enjoy your new teeth for a week or two until the retainer is ready.

Retainers

Retainers are removable appliances, meaning that you can put them in and take them out at will. Of course, the orthodontist will want you to wear them the greater part of each day and all night, but you can take them out to brush your teeth or eat a meal.

Upper and lower retainers are quite different. The upper one contains more acrylic because it nestles against the roof of your mouth. Wire set into the acrylic maintains the spaces between certain teeth, as you can see from the illustration. Wire attached to each side of the retainer extends around the front teeth. Like the archwire, this wire will keep your teeth from moving back.

The lower retainer has less acrylic because your tongue lies in the bottom of your mouth. The acrylic follows the tooth line, pushing snugly against the teeth. The wire attached to each end extends around the front of the teeth. You will feel pressure when you first insert the retainer, but that pressure is needed to keep the teeth from moving back to their original positions. After a day or so, you'll get used to the feeling and won't notice any pressure. It will feel snug only when you first pop it into your mouth.

Here's the fun part about retainers: you can get the acrylic in any color you want. I've seen blue retainers and red retainers and even multicolored retainers. Of course, no one will see the color unless you take the retainers out to show, but they're fun to have anyway. I've even seen retainers with the wearer's initials designed into them.

Along with the retainers, you'll be given a carrying case for them. Be sure to keep the retainers in the case when you're not wearing them, because they are easily damaged. The case keeps them secure and free from germs. You can even get a colored case so that it stands out when you're looking for it.

Eating with Retainers

You won't want to eat while wearing your retainers. Most people figure this out, but my orthodontist made such a big deal about my wearing the retainers all the time that I thought I was supposed to eat with them in place.

The first time I tried that in the school cafeteria, bread from my sandwich stuck to the retainer on the roof of my mouth. I tried washing the bread down with milk, but that only made the bread cling more tenaciously.

I excused myself from the table and dashed to the restroom. My plan was to wash the retainer in the sink and get all that bread off. But when I arrived, several girls stood in front of the sink combing their hair. They were popular girls, too; I certainly didn't want them to see me pull out my retainers with food stuck all over them.

I stood there, debating what to do. Minutes ticked by; first lunch was almost over. I worked my way to the sink, but because the girls didn't leave, I decided against rinsing my retainers. I washed my hands instead, and then went back to the cafeteria. The piece of cake I ate stuck to my retainer, too.

During my next class, I asked permission to go to the restroom, where I finally washed my retainers in private. They looked fine after I rinsed the bread and cake off them.

I went through that process for a whole year; it never dawned on me to take the retainers out before eating. I guess I was embarrassed about removing them in front of anyone, but retainers aren't false teeth. There's nothing wrong with removing them discreetly. If you're afraid you'll drool when you pull them out (and that sometimes happens), simply turn aside and take them out. Or go to the bathroom and do it. So many people are wearing braces nowadays, and then retainers, that retainers are commonplace.

Cleaning Your Retainers

Your retainers, like your teeth, need daily cleaning. Rinsing is not enough; you'll want to give them a thorough cleaning to rid them of germs and plaque. My dental hygienist suggested using a liquid antibacterial soap to clean the retainers. Simply pour a little liquid soap on them and use a toothbrush to brush over the acrylic. Rinse carefully and make sure nothing is clinging to the wire.

Treat your retainers carefully, and they will last as long as they're needed. Keep them clean, and you'll see that food doesn't cling to them and decay in your mouth.

Problems with Retainers

Problems may crop up because retainers are removable appliances. You didn't lose your braces because they were

Branches 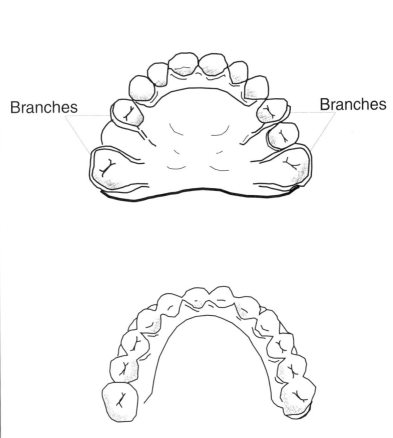 **Branches**

Upper and lower retainers.

attached to your teeth. However, retainers have ways of getting lost, thrown away, stolen, and eaten.

Kathy and Starr had been shopping at the mall one afternoon. They were hungry, they stopped to get a bite to eat at one of the fast-food shops in the food court. Starr carefully popped her retainers out. Not wanting to gross out anyone who might be looking, she discreetly folded them in a napkin and set them beside her food tray.

82

The girls giggled their way through their meal. Then a couple of their classmates who worked in the food court came over to sit with them.

The girls chatted even longer. Finally, Kathy looked at her watch and said, "Wow, it's almost 5:00. I was supposed to be home with the car by 5:30." She grabbed her trash and threw it into the can.

Starr was playing with one last french fry. She put it in her mouth and piled her trash on her food tray— including the napkin that was wrapped around her retainers. Then she dumped it all into the trash can.

As the girls got into Kathy's car, Starr realized she wasn't wearing her retainers. She quickly went through her purse and found the case. Empty.

"Oh, no," she said. "I don't have my retainers."

Kathy thought a moment. "Did you have them when we ate?"

"I took them out," Starr said. "I wrapped them in a napkin and put them by my tray."

"What did you do with the napkin?"

Starr looked sick. "I threw everything away," she said.

When you take your retainers out and wrap them in a napkin, it's easy to confuse them with trash. Before you realize it, you've thrown them out, and you may not think about it again until you're miles away from that particular trash can.

Your first retainers are part of the cost your parents have already paid for the braces. But you have to pay separately for any replacements. Retainers cost about $100.

To be safe, it's best to put your retainers in the case whenever you take them out of your mouth. Put the case in your pocket or bag. Or at least, leave the case out on the table where it won't be mixed up with the trash.

Sometimes kids steal others' retainers. At my daughter's school, kids have to be careful when they put their retainers down, even in the case, because other kids may walk off with them. Teachers have lamented that stealing retainers is the latest fad, whether it's because kids know they're a hassle to replace or because it's a status act. My daughter lost her retainers when she put them in the case on her desk to eat some candy the teacher had handed out. By the end of class, the case had disappeared from her desk.

Chewable Toys for Pets
Retainers also get eaten. Not by people, of course, but pets apparently love to sink their teeth into the acrylic. According to my dentist, the retainer has just the right feel for a cat or small dog. If you leave a retainer on the table, it can either fall on the floor (where your pet will find it in no time), or your cat may jump up on the table and make a meal out of it right then and there.

Again, to prevent something like this from happening, get in the habit of storing your retainers in the case every time you take them out of your mouth.

Embarrassing Yourself
Another reason to store your retainers in the case is to avoid embarrassing yourself. Someone else's retainer lying loose on the dinner table is not an appealing sight.

Sheryl and her friends sat down to eat with some of their classmates. Sheryl found herself next to a guy in her math class. She'd always found him attractive, but was too shy to talk to him.

As she continued to talk to her girlfriends, she tried to edge closer to Daniel to include him in their conversation.

She moved her hand closer and closer to his plate.

Suddenly, one of her friends shrieked, "What's that? Oh, gross." She was pointing to Daniel's retainers that were lying uncovered right beside Sheryl's hand.

Sheryl jerked her hand away when Amelia screamed.

Another guy noticed Daniel's retainers and grabbed one, shooting it across the table to the girl who'd screamed.

"Ewww," she said.

Daniel jumped up to retrieve his retainer; he stuck the other one into the pocket of his jeans. His face was beet-red. Sheryl tried to think of something to say, but all she kept picturing was that gross retainer lying on the table by her hand. And she'd almost touched it!

Maybe you don't think your retainers are particularly gross, and they aren't. However, to someone else, it's unappealing (to say the least) to find them lying uncovered on the dining room table, or on the coffee table in the living room. If you don't want to upset anyone else (and who knows when your Aunt Lucy is going to drop by?), keep the retainer in the case. It's just good manners.

Nervous Habits with Retainers

Retainers are supposed to fit snugly in your mouth, but

after a while you can use your tongue to pop one out. Popping out a retainer can become a nervous habit, and before you know it, you can pop one out when you don't mean to. Don't worry; you can't really send it flying across a room, but you will no doubt annoy people by flicking it around in your mouth.

Your retainers help to maintain the corrections the orthodontist has made to your teeth. But they have to be worn most of the time in order to do their job. Because they're easy to remove, be careful not to end up removing them more than you wear them. Which leads to the matter of compliance.

Compliance with Appointments

Your appointments with the orthodontist don't end once your braces are removed. You still need to go back periodically for checkups, so that the orthodontist can determine how well your retainers are working out. But you don't have to go as frequently as before—usually every three months.

Be sure to take your retainers with you to every appointment. Your orthodontist will want to check their fit and see if you need new retainers made. Sometimes he'll only tighten the wire; sometimes he may make a new impression of your teeth and then another retainer.

How soon you can stop wearing your retainers has a lot to do with how compliant you are with treatment. If you wear your retainers according to the orthodontist's instructions, you'll make faster progress than the patient who wears her retainer only every once in a while.

If you stop wearing your retainers regularly, you'll find it harder to remember to wear them at all. Not wearing the retainers can allow your teeth to shift out of their new positions.

Missing appointments and then forgetting to make another one for a month or so can also lead to problems. Compliance means keeping your appointments and following the orthodontist's instructions. Before you know it, your retainers will have done their work, and your days in braces and retainers will be only a distant memory.

Afterword

I have tried to paint as reassuring a picture of the braces' experience as I could. Reality these days means that many of you are going to go to the orthodontist, and many of you will wear braces and other appliances for two or three years. Techniques have changed so much, and braces have become such a common experience, that you shouldn't feel intimidated or alone.

Having braces can be as good an experience as you let it be. The better informed you are, the less afraid you'll be. My hope is that this book has given you an idea how important braces are in correcting a number of problems commonly faced by teens.

All the teenagers I spoke with were pleased with the end result; they were also quick to forget how uncomfortable certain procedures had been or how inconvenient those monthly appointments were. Braces became a transforming part of their adolescence, and most teens came away from the experience with improved self-esteem.

Braces also taught my daughter a valuable lesson: one that wound up in her high school's memory book. "I've learned so far," Stevie wrote in her sophomore year, "that you really can't die of embarrassment."

Although braces and retainers may offer a few embarrassing moments, those times will fade. Your perfect smile will not.

Glossary

archwire Wire attached to braces to exert force on the teeth to move them.

articular disc Tissue separating the jawbone from the condyle.

bands Plastic or metal pieces that encircle the teeth and hold brackets.

brackets The part of braces from which tie rings attach the archwire to the teeth.

condyle Bony, knoblike protuberance at the end of the bone to which the facial muscles are attached in the jawbone.

cross bite Improper meeting of the teeth where the difference between upper and lower teeth is from side to side.

flat plane splint Removable mouthpiece that prevents gnashing of the teeth. The splint is smooth on the surface presenting to the opposing teeth.

headgear Removable parts of braces that attach to the teeth and wrap around the wearer's head.

malocclusion An improper bite.

mandible The lower jawbone.

orthodontist Dentist who specializes in correcting crooked and poorly aligned teeth.

overbite Vertical overlapping of the lower teeth by the upper teeth.

palate spreader Mouthpiece installed in the roof of the mouth to widen the arch.

repositioning splint Removable mouthpiece to prevent the grinding or gnashing of teeth. The surface presenting to the opposing teeth is indented to reposition the teeth in its bite.

retainer Removable mouthpiece that holds the teeth in place after repositioning by braces.

space maintainer Mouthpiece, similar to a retainer, that holds space open for a new tooth.

TMJ Temporomandibular joint syndrome, characterized by facial muscle pain, misaligned teeth, headaches, and joint pain.

Where to Go for Help

American Association of Orthodontists
401 North Lindbergh Boulevard
St. Louis, MO 63141
(314) 993-1700 phone
(314) 997-1745 fax
E-mail: info@aaortho.org
Web site: http://www.aaortho.org/

American Board of Orthodontics
401 North Lindbergh Boulevard
St. Louis, MO 63141
(314) 432-6130 phone

Dental Bytes Magazine
Web site: http://www.dentalbytes.com/

The Orthodontic Information Page
Web site: http://www.bracesinfo.com/

Webdental: The Dental Database
Web site: http://www.webdental.com/html/orthodontics.shtml

For Further Reading

Betancourt, Jeanne. *Smile! How to Cope with Braces.* New York: Alfred A. Knopf, 1982.

Catalano, Ellen Mohr, and Kimeron Hardin. *The Chronic Pain Control Workbook.* Oakland, CA: New Harbinger Publications, 1996.

Foster, Malcolm S. *Protecting Our Children's Teeth.* New York: Plenum Press, 1992.

Gibilisco, Joseph, Charles McNeill, and Harold Perry. *Orofacial Pain.* Carol Stream, IL: Quintessence Co., Inc., 1994.

Goldstein, Ronald. *Change Your Smile.* Chicago: Quintessence Pub. Co., Inc., 1984.

Kaplan, Andrew, and Gray Williams, Jr. *The TMJ Book.* New York: Pharos Books, 1988.

Kroeger, Robert. *How to Overcome Fear of Dentistry.* Cincinnati; Heritage Communications, 1988.

Moles, Randall C. *Ending Head and Neck Pain.* Racine, WI: CGM Publications, 1989.

Stay, Flora Parsa. *The Complete Book of Dental Remedies.* Garden City Park, NY: Avery Publishing Group, 1995.

Index